PHARMACEUTICAL

DISPENSING

W0193406

PHARMACEUTICAL

DISPENSING

Pratibha Nand
M. Pharm. (Pharmaceutics)
Lecturer, Maharaja Surajmal Institute of
Pharmacy and Technology, New Delhi

Roop K. Khar
M. Pharm., D.B.M., Ph.D. (Sofia)
Head, Deptt. of Pharmaceutics,
Hamdard University, New Delhi

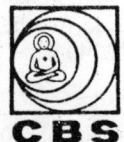

CBS

CBS Publishers & Distributors Pvt. Ltd.

New Delhi • Bengaluru • Chennai • Kochi • Kolkata • Mumbai
Hyderabad • Nagpur • Patna • Pune • Vijayawada

ISBN: 81-239-0394-4

First Edition: 1995
Reprint: 2002, 2004, 2006, 2007, 2010,
      2014, 2017, 2018, 2019

Copyright © Publisher

All rights reserved. No part of this book may be reproduced or transmitted in any form or by any means, electronic or mechanical, including photocopying, recording, or any information storage and retrieval system without permission, in writing, from the publisher.

Published by **Satish Kumar Jain** and produced by **Varun Jain** for
CBS Publishers & Distributors Pvt. Ltd.,
4819/XI Prahlad Street, 24 Ansari Road, Daryaganj, New Delhi - 110002
delhi@cbspd.com, cbspubs@airtelmail.in • www.cbspd.com
Ph.: 23289259, 23266861, 23266867 • Fax: 011-23243014

Corporate Office: 204 FIE, Industrial Area, Patparganj, Delhi - 110 092
Ph: 49344934 • Fax: 011-49344935
E-mail: publishing@cbspd.com • publicity@cbspd.com

Branches:
• *Bengaluru:* 2975, 17th Cross, K.R. Road, Bansankari 2nd Stage,
  Bengaluru - 70 • Ph: +91-80-26771678/79 • Fax: +91-80-26771680
  E-mail: cbsbng@gmail.com, bangalore@cbspd.com
• *Chennai:* No. 7, Subbaraya Street, Shenoy Nagar, Chennai - 600030
  Ph: +91-44-26681266, 26680620 • Fax: +91-44-42032115
  E-mail: chennai@cbspd.com
• *Kochi:* Ashana House, 39/1904, A.M. Thomas Road, Valanjambalam,
  Ernakulum, Kochi • Ph: +91-484-4059061-65
  Fax: +91-484-4059065 • E-mail: cochin@cbspd.com
• *Kolkata:* 6-B, Ground Floor, Rameshwar Shaw Road, Kolkata - 700014
  Ph: +91-33-22891126/7/8 • E-mail: kolkata@cbspd.com
• *Mumbai:* 83-C, Dr. E. Moses Road, Worli, Mumbai - 400018
  Ph: +91-9833017933, 022-24902340/41 • E-mail: mumbai@cbspd.com

Representatives:

• Hyderabad: 0-9885175004	• Nagpur: 0-9021734563
• Patna: 0-9334159340	• Pune: 0-9623451994
• Jharkhand: 0-9811541605	• Uttarakhand: 0-9716462459

Printed at:
Neekunj Print Process, Delhi (India)

Preface

The role of dispensing pharmacy has undergone tremendous changes in last few decades. In order to match the need of the hour, various universities have changed their syllabi to satisfy the new requirements. Many are in the process of doing do. Similarly at the Diploma Pharmacy level Pharmacy Council of India has come up with new regulations which have been made effective throughout the country.

It is with this intention that the authors undertook the present task, to make reading material available to the students of Pharmacy. First three chapters deal with basics in dispensing pharmacy like prescription, incompatibilities and posology. Following five chapters from 4th to 8th describe various common dosage forms in dispensing practice. Ninth chapter discusses various commonly used cosmetic formulations. The tenth and eleventh chapters go through various aspects of sterile dosage forms and ophthalmic products. A brief introduction and formulation aspects of tablets and capsules have been dealt with in chapters 12 and 13. To assist the students and the teachers alike, there are various appendices which deal with common topics like drug interactions, pharmaceutical calculations, revision questions and patent and proprietary products.

PRATIBHA NAND
ROOP K. KHAR

Acknowledgement

At the outset we would like to express our thanks to our families for their immense cooperation in undertaking and completing this project. We would not have reached our goal had it not been for the guidance, co-operation and inspiration of Seema, Arvind, Rachna and Nirmal. We also express our thanks to our colleagues. Finally we thank our publishers for their unfailing consideration and patience.

Contents

1

Prescription

Definition

Prescription is an order written by a physician, dentist or any other registered medical practitioner to a pharmacist to compound and dispense a specific medication for the patient.

Parts of a Prescription

A prescription consists of following parts :

1. Date
2. Name, age, sex and address of the patient
3. Superscription
4. Inscription
5. Subscription
6. Signatura
7. Signature, address, registration No. of the prescriber.

1. Date

Date on the prescription helps a pharmacist for controlling the supply of narcotic drugs. It is also useful when a prescription is brought for dispensing long time after its issue.

2. Name, age, sex and address of the patient

These particulars avoid the possibility of giving the finished product to a person other than the one it is meant for. It helps in checking the medication and dose especially in case of children.

3. Superscription

It is represented by a symbol Rx which is always written at the top left hand corner. In the earlier days of superstition, the symbol was considered as a prayer to Jupiter, God of healing, but now it is understood as an abbreviation of Latin term recipe, meaning 'take thou' or 'you take'.

4. Inscription

This is the main part of prescription. It consists of a list of ingredients, and the quantity of each that is to be used.

5. Subscription

This part contains prescriber's directions to the pharmacist regarding the dosage form to be prepared and No. of doses to be dispensed.

6. Signatura

It is usually abbreviated as 'sig.' on the prescriptions and consists of the directions to be given to the patient regarding the administration of the drug.

7. Signature, address and registration number of prescriber

The prescriptions containing narcotic or other habit-forming drugs must bear the address and registration number of the prescriber. This gives the special identification and authenticates the prescription.

Reading and Understanding of Prescription

1. Receiving

The prescription should be received from the patient by the pharmacist himself. No unauthorised person should try to receive or read the prescription.

2. Reading and checking

(i) The prescription should be read in the dispensing room or laboratory where there will be no disturbance for the pharmacist.

(ii) All abbreviations in the prescription should be properly understood. If necessary, the pharmacist should not hesitate to consult his colleagues. If there is still ambiguity, the prescriber should be contacted for clarification. As number of drugs are available in the market, mistakes occur due to similarity of pronunciation and spellings. Examples of such drugs which look alike or sound alike are given below :

Doriden	Doxidan
Digoxin	Digitoxin
Prednisone	Prednisolone
Marax	Atarax

(iii) If there is any omission of any important particular such as the dose, the prescriber should be contacted.

(iv) The size and frequency of the dose must be carefully verified and checked.

3. Pricing of prescription

The prescription should be priced immediately after receiving it and the patient informed of it. This should be done before starting the compounding of prescription so that there will not be any dispute.

4. Marking the prescription

The prescription is marked with a rubber stamp to indicate that it has been dispensed.

5. Labelling

The label is written before dispensing the prescription so as to prevent the dispensing of an excessive dose, since the label states the strength of preparation supplied and the actual amount that the patient has to take at a particular time.

Table 1.1. Latin terms and abbreviations

Latin term	Abbreviation	English meaning
Quantum sufficiat/ Quantum sufficit	q.s.	As much as is sufficient
Ad	aa, aa	Up to
Ana	aa, aa	Of each
Parte aequals	pt. aeq.	Equal parts
Auristillae	auristill	Ear drops
Capsula	caps.	A capsule
Amylacea	amylac.	A cachet
Cataplasma	cataplasm.	A poultice
Charta	chart.	A powder
Collunarium	collun.	A nose wash
Collutorium	collut.	A mouth wash
Collyrium	collyr.	An eye lotion
Cremor	crem.	A cream
Emulsio	emul.	An emulsion
Guttae	gtt.	Drops
Haustus	ht.	A draught
Inhalatio	inhal.	An inhalation

Contd.

Latin term	Abbreviation	English meaning
Injectio	inj.	An injection
Insufflatio	insuff.	An insufflation
Linimentum	lin.	A liniment
Liquor	liq.	A solution
Lotio	lot.	A lotion
Mistura	m., mist.	A mixture
Naristillae	narist.	Nasal drops
Nebula	neb.	A spray
Oblatum	oblat.	A cachet
Oculentum	oculent.	An eye ointment
Pasta	past.	A paste
Pilula	pil.	A pill
Pulvis	pulv.	A powder
Pulvis conspersus	pulv. consper.	A dusting powder
Solvellae	solv.	Solution tablets
Sternutamentum	sternut.	A snuff
Supporsitorium	suppos.	A suppository
Tabella/Tabletta	tab.	A tablet
Unguentum	ung.	An ointment
Vapor	vap.	An inhalation
Adde, Addatur	add.	Add. Let (it) be added
Divide, Dividatur	div.	Divide. Let (it) be divided
Dividatur in aequales	div. in pt. aeq.	Divide into equal parts
Fiat	ft.	Let (it) be made
Fiant	ft.	Let (them) be made
Misce, Misceatur	m.	Mix. Let (it) be mixed
Misce fiat mistura	m. ft. m.	Mix to make a mixture
Misce secundum artem	m.s.a.	Mix pharmaceutically
Duplum	duplum	Twice the quantity
Inphiala	—	In a bottle
Mitte mitt	mitt.	Send
Phiala prius agiata	p.p.a.	The bottle being first shaken
Talis, Tales	tal.	Such
Addendus	addend.	To be added
Applicandus	applicand.	To be applied
Applicat	—	Let (him) apply
Applicetur	applicat.	Let (it) be applied

Contd.

Latin term	Abbreviation	English meaning
Capiendus	capiend.	To be taken
Infricandus	infricand.	To be rubbed in
Inhaletur	inhal.	Let (it) be inhaled
Instillandus	instilland.	To be dropped in
Miscendus	miscend.	To be mixed
Signa	sig.	Label
Summendus	s. or sum.	To be taken
Utendus	u. or utend.	To be used
Ad libitum	ad. lib.	As much as you please
Dimidium	dimid.	The half
Dosis	dos.	A dose
Guttatim	guttatim	Drop by drop
Mensura	mens.	By measure
Pro	pro	For
Pro dosi	—	As a dose

Time of administration or application

(a) Times per day

Semel in die	sem. in die	Once a day
Bis in die, Bis die	b.i.d., b.d.	Twice a day
Ter in die, Ter die	t.i.d., t.d.	Three times a day
Quater in die	q.i.d., q.d.	Four times a day
Sexies in die	sex in d.	Six times a day
Bis terve in die	b.t.i.d.	Two or three times a day
Ter quaterve die	t.q.d.	Three or four times a day
Quotidie	quot.	Daily
Ter quotidie	ter quot.	Three times daily

(b) Parts of the day

Primo mane	prim. m.	Early in the morning
Mane	m.	In the morning
Omni mane	o.m.	Every morning
Jentaculum	jentac.	Breakfast
Nocte	n.	At night
Inter noctem	inter noct.	During the night
Omni nocte	o.n.	Every night

Contd.

Latin term	*Abbreviation*	*English meaning*
Hora somni	h.s.	At bedtime
Nocte et mane	n. et m.	Night and morning
Nocte maneque	n.m.	Night and morning
Hac nocte	hac noct.	Tonight

(c) Hour time

Omni hora, Quaque hora	o.h., qq.h.	Every hour
Omni quarta hora, Quaque quarta hora	o.q.h., qq.q.h.	Every fourth hour
Singulis horis	sing. hor.	Every hour
Alternis horis	alt. hor.	Every two hours
Tertis horis	tert. hor.	Every three hours
Quartis horis	quart. hor.	Every four hours
Sextis horis	sext. hor.	Every six hours

(d) Correlated time

Ante cibos	a.c.	Before meals
Post cibos	p.c.	After meals
Inter cibos	i.c.	Between meals

(e) Other terms

Dolore urgente	dol. urg.	When the pain is severe
More dicto	m.d.	As directed
Modo dicto	m.d.	As directed
Pro re nata	p.r.n.	Occasionally
Quoties opus sit	quot. o.s.	As often as necessary
Si dolor urgeat	si dol. urg.	If the pain is severe
Si opus sit	s.o.s.	When required
Statim	stat.	Immediately. At once
Tussi urgente	tuss. urg.	If the cough is troublesome
Cum	c.	With
Cum duplo	c. dup.	With twice as much
Cum parte aequale	c. pt. aeq.	With an equal quantity
Cum tanto	c. tant.	With as much
Cyathus	cyath.	A glass
Cyathus vinousus	cyath. vin.	A wineglass

Contd.

Latin term	Abbreviation	English meaning
E lacte	e lact.	With milk
Ex aqua	ex aq.	With water
Dexter	dext.	Right
Laevus	laev.	Left
Parti affectae applicandus	p.a.a.	To be applied on the affected part
Partibus affectis	p.a.	To the affected parts
Sinister	sinist.	Left
Auri	auri	To the ear
Naso	—	To the throat
Oculis	ocul.	For the eyes
Pro oculils	pro ocul.	For the eyes

Numerals

Arabic	Roman	
No.	Symbol	Cardinal
1	I	unus
2	II	duo
3	III	tres ter
4	IV	quattuor or quatuor
5	V	quinque quinquies
6	VI	sex
7	VII	septem
8	VIII	octo
9	IX	novem
10	X	decem
11	XI	undecim
12	XII	duodecim
14	XIV	quattuordecim
15	XV	quindecim
20	XX	viginti
50	L	quinquaginta
100	C	centum, centies

Modern Methods of Prescribing

Prescription writing has now been changed due to several developments. Nowadays preparations are generally compounded by pharmaceutical companies and the pharmacist's role is dispensing and advising patients about quantity, drug interactions, adverse reactions, etc.

There are four types of prescriptions :

1. Hospital prescriptions for 'in patients'
2. Hospital prescriptions for 'out patients'
3. Prescriptions in general practice
4. Private prescriptions

In general, a prescription should be precise, accurate, clear and readable. The practice of writing long, complicated prescriptions containing many active ingredients, adjuvants, vehicles has now been changed. Today pharmaceutical companies provide combinations of several ingredients.

A drug may be prescribed by its non-proprietary or official (generic) name or proprietary (brand or trade) name. There are certain advantages and disadvantages of writing a prescription by their proprietary names which are mentioned below :

Advantages

1. Proprietary names are easy to remember and catchy, e.g., Librium (Chlordiazepoxide).
2. They provide ease in communication with the patient.
3. For some drugs a change in tablet adjuvants provide important effects on the absorption of drug from the formulation.
4. Continuity can be achieved by prescribing the same proprietary name every time.

Disadvantages

1. Pharmacist cannot legally dispense the substitute of the drug which is present in stocks.
2. It is cheaper to prescribe the drugs by official name.

Hence it is clear that in hospitals drugs should be prescribed by non-proprietary names so that the pharmacist can dispense the formulation which is in stock. In general practice, prescriber can use proprietary name.

Modern methods of prescription writing eliminate the use of Latin terms. These were used in the past to conceal from the patient, the nature of a drug. Nowadays, the prescriptions are written in English. Further it is also advisable to state the dose in milligrams instead of using the decimal fraction of a gram.

Prescription Writing for Controlled Drugs

These drugs can be categorised into three classes :

1. Class A : morphine, pethidine, LSD, cocaine, diamorphine
2. Class B : codeine, cannabis, oral amphetamines
3. Class C : benzphetamine, chlorphentermine, pipradrol

Prescriptions for above mentioned categories must include :

1. Date, signature
2. Prescriber's address
3. Prescriber's own handwriting
4. Name and address of patient
5. Total quantity of drug or number of doses in both words and figures
6. Exact dose in both words and figures

If the prescription does not follow these instructions the pharmacist shall not dispense it.

A typical prescription

ROHINI HOSPITAL
A-1, Avantika Road
Telephone : 7271898

Name : Mr. Amit   *Date :* June 26, 1994
Address : 203, Anand Vihar   *Age :* 30

Tetracycline, 250 mg capsules. Dispense twenty.
Label : Take one capsule with water four times a day
for 5 days.

Refills _____   *Signature* _____
     Regd. No. _____
     Dispense as written _____
     Substitution permitted _____

ADOPTION OF METRIC SYSTEM

Metrology is defined as science of measurements and weights. There are two systems for weights and measurements.

1. **Imperial system.** It is an old system based on unrelated units, e.g., grains, drachms, ounce and gallons.
2. **Metric system or decimal system.** It is based on related units, e.g., milligrams, grams, centimetres, metres.

Measures of Weight

Standard unit of mass (weight) is kilograms and all other units of mass are derived from kilogram.

1 kilogram (kg)	=	1000 g
1 hectogram (hg)	=	100 g
1 decagram (dag)	=	10 g
1 gram (gm)	=	1 g
1 decigram (dg)	=	0.1 g = 100 mg
1 centigram (cg)	=	0.01 g = 10 mg
1 milligram (mg)	=	0.001 g = 1 mg
1 microgram (μg or mcg)	=	1/1000 mg

Measures of Capacity

Standard unit for measures of capacity is litre and all other measures of capacity are derived from it.

     1 litre (lt)   =   1000 ml

The calculation in metric system is simple. In Imperial system the weight and volume of water are not numerically equal quantities as in metric system. At 4°C, 1 g of water measures 1 ml whereas 1 grain of water measures 1.1 minims. Similarly 437.5 grains (1 oz) of water measures 480 minims at 16.7°C and 460.2 minims at 4°C. If 1 grain is present in 1.1 minims or 437.5 grains are present in 1 fl oz, the solution would have same concentration as 1 g in 1 ml.

This system provides easier calculation, greater accuracy and flexibility. It is widely used system by official agencies. For many years, the British Pharmacopoeia Commission has been advocating the use of metric system in prescribing. The B.P. 1963 has adopted the use of metric system and has abandoned the use of Imperial system completely. Single dose drug preparations like tablets, capsules, injections and similar preparations are available only in metric dose forms. B.P. Commission has published a schedule of metric/Imperial equivalent doses. Thus, when a half grain tablet is prescribed the pharmacist may supply 30 mg tablet.

CALCULATIONS INVOLVED IN DISPENSING

1. *Rx*

Heavy magnesium carbonate	6.00 g
Light magnesium carbonate	6.00 g
Rhubarb powder	6.00 g
Ginger powder	2.00 g

Make powder, send 100 g.

Calculation : To get the required quantities for 100 g, multiply the given quantity by 5.

2. *Rx*

Atropine sulphate   1/120 gr

Mix to make powder. Send such five.

Rule : Calculate for one extra powder.

Quantity for 6 powders $= \dfrac{1}{120} \times 6 = 1/20$ gr

To remove this fraction we will add 19 grains of lactose.

1 grain of atropine sulphate + 19 grains of lactose

$$= 20 \text{ grains of powder}$$

$$= \frac{19 + 1}{20} = \frac{20}{20} = 1 \text{ gr.} \qquad \text{... Drug admixture (A)}$$

But we cannot weigh less than 2 grains. Therefore total quantity required for 6 powders $= 2 \times 6 = 12$ grains.

1 grain of drug admixture (A) is already with us so $(12 - 1 =)$ 11 gr of lactose should be added to make it 12 gr.

1 gr of drug admixture (A) + 11 gr of lactose = 12 gr

                                               ... Drug admixture (B)

3. Percentage calculation

(i) *Weight in volume (w/v) solutions*

In this 1 g solute is dissolved in sufficient amount of water to produce 100 ml to make 1% w/v.

Solid	1 part by weight
Solvent	100 parts by volume

(ii) *Weight in weight (w/w) solutions*

In this the solute and the solvent are taken by weight. The general formula for 1% w/w solution is

Solid	1 part by weight

Solvent to produce   100 parts by weight

(iii) *Volume by volume (v/v) solutions*

In this the solute and solvent are taken by volume. The general formula
for 1% v/v solution is

Solute   1 part by volume
Solvent to produce   100 parts by volume

General formula (points to be remembered)

1. If the numerical has metric system as unit of measurement and
    only one percentage is given then follow the following formula :

$$\text{Quantity of solute required} = \frac{1}{100} \times P \times Q$$

where P = percentage required

Q = quantity required.

2. 1 fl. oz of 1% w/v solution requires 4.375 grains of solute.

    1 gallon of 1% solution requires 700 grains of solute.

    If the numerical has imperial system as a unit of measurement
    and only one percentage is given then follow this general
    formula :

$$\text{Quantity of solute required} = \frac{35}{8} \times P \times Q = 4.375 \times P \times Q$$

where P = percentage required

Q = quantity required.

3. Volume of stronger solution to be used

$$= \frac{\text{volume required} \times \text{percentage required}}{\text{percentage used}}$$

Examples

1. How will you prepare 50 ml of 5% solution of sodium chloride?

Ans. Quantity of sodium chloride $= \dfrac{1}{100} \times P \times Q$

$$= \frac{1}{100} \times 5 \times 50 = 2.5 \text{ g.}$$

2. How will you prepare 8 fluid ounce of 5% solution of mercuric
    chloride?

Ans. Quantity of mercuric chloride $= \dfrac{35}{8} \times P \times Q$

$$= \frac{35}{8} \times 5 \times 8$$

$= 175$ grains   [1 grain = 65 mg]

$= 175 \times 65 = 11.37$ g

Quantity of water = 8 fl oz = 8 × 30   [1 fl oz = 30 ml]

$\qquad\qquad\qquad = 240$ ml

3. How will you prepare 2 fl oz of glucose of 5% concentration?

Ans. Quantity of glucose = $4.375 \times P \times Q = 4.375 \times 5 \times 2 = 43.75$ gr

$\qquad\qquad\qquad\qquad = 43.75 \times 65$ [1 grain = 65 mg]

$\qquad\qquad\qquad\qquad = 2.84$ g

Quantity of water = 2 fl oz = 2 × 30 = 60 ml.

4. How will you prepare 2 fl oz of 4% of acetic acid from 33% acetic acid?

Ans. Vol. of real acetic acid required for dilution

$$= \frac{\text{volume required} \times \text{percentage required}}{\text{percentage used}}$$

$$= \frac{2 \times 4}{33} = \frac{8}{33} = 0.24 \text{ fl oz} = 0.24 \times 30 = 7.2 \text{ ml.}$$

So quantity of water = 60 – 7.2 = 52.8 ml   [2 fl oz = 60 ml]

4. Alligation method

It involves mixing of two similar preparations but of different strengths to produce a preparation of intermediate strength.

A. Alligation medial

This is used to calculate the percentage strength of a mixture that has been made by mixing two or more components of given percentage strengths.

Example : What is the percentage of zinc oxide in an ointment prepared by mixing 200 g of 10% ointment, 50 g of 20% ointment, and 100 g of 5% ointment?

Solution :

10	×	200	=	2000
20	×	50	=	1000
5	×	100	=	500
Total :		350		3500

Percentage of zinc oxide $= \dfrac{3500}{350} = 10\%$

In solving such problems, following steps are to be followed :

1. Determine the total amount of active ingredient and the total amount of mixture.
2. Multiply the strength by amount and add the products and divide by the sum of amounts to give the strength of the mixture.

B. *Alligation alternate*

This method is used to find relative amounts of solution or other substances of different strength, that should be mixed to make a mixture of required strength. A substance with higher value than that required can easily be expected to be in low amount and vice versa. The gain in value or loss in amount of one substance always balances the loss in value or gain in amount of another substance. It is also called the 'method of rectangles'.

Rules :

1. Known strengths are to be put on the left hand corners of a rectangle and the required strengths are at the point of intersection of diagonals.
2. The figure with a smaller value can be subtracted from larger figure on the same diagonal and the result is written at the other end.
3. Values of the other end of the horizontal line indicates the parts of the respective substances to be mixed.

Example : In what proportion 30% alcohol and 95% alcohol be mixed to make 500 ml of 50% alcohol.

Solution :

Thus 20 parts of 95% alcohol and 45 parts of 30% alcohol should be mixed to get 65 parts.

$$65 : 500 \text{ ml} : : 20 \text{ parts} : x \text{ ml}$$

$$x = \frac{500 \times 20}{65} = 154 \text{ ml.}$$

Amount of 30% alcohol can be calculated by subtracting 154 ml from 500 ml.

$$\begin{array}{lll} \text{Total amount} & = 500 \text{ ml} \\ \underline{95\% \text{ alcohol}} & \underline{= 154 \text{ ml}} \\ 30\% \text{ alcohol} & = 346 \text{ ml} \end{array}$$

Example : In what proportion should we mix 50%, 20% and 5% zinc oxide to produce 10% ointment?

Solution :

1. Write the percentage strength in descending order on the L.H.S. of vertical line and required percentage in between the two vertical lines.
2. Two lots containing more (50% and 20%) than the desired percentage may be separately linked to the lot containing less (5%) than the desired percentages.
3. Subtract the required strength from the higher strength and write the values horizontally against the lowest strength on R.H.S.
4. The sum of two values indicates the parts of the lowest strength required.
5. Subtract the lowest strength from the required strength and put the remainder on the right hand side.

50%		5 parts of 50% ointment
20%	10	5 parts of 20% ointment
5%		10 + 40 = 50 parts of 5% ointment

Relative amounts   5 : 5 : 50   or   1 : 1 : 10

$$\begin{array}{rcccc} 50 & \times & 1 & = & 50 \\ 20 & \times & 1 & = & 20 \\ 5 & \times & 10 & = & 50 \\ \hline \text{Total :} & & 12 & & 120 \\ \hline \end{array}$$

Percentage of zinc oxide $= \dfrac{120}{12} = 10\%$

Example : How many parts of 20%, 15%, 5% and 3% alcohol should be mixed to get 10% ointment?

Solution :

20%		7 parts of 20% ointment
15%	10	5 parts of 15% ointment
5%		5 parts of 5% ointment
3%		10 parts of 3% ointment

Relative amounts   7 : 5 : 5 : 10

$$
\begin{array}{rcrcr}
20 & \times & 7 & = & 140 \\
15 & \times & 5 & = & 75 \\
5 & \times & 5 & = & 25 \\
3 & \times & 10 & = & 30 \\
\hline
\text{Total :} & & 27 & & 270 \\
\hline
\end{array}
$$

Percentage of alcohol $= \dfrac{270}{27} = 10\%$

5. Displacement value of medicaments for suppositories

Suppositories for their preparation require :

  (i) medicament

  (ii) base.

Displacement value is considered for suppositories because the density of these two is not the same. Therefore, it becomes necessary to calculate the displacement value of medicament to ensure its correct amount in suppositories.

Definition

Displacement value can be defined as the amount of medicament which displaces one part of the standard base used. Generally theobroma oil is used as a base. When glycero-gelatin base is used, density factor 1.2 should be taken into consideration.

The displacement values of some commonly used medicaments are given in Table No. 8.1.

Example : Prepare 8 suppositories each containing 300 mg of bismuth subgallate. The displacement value of bismuth subgallate is 3.

Ans. To take wastage into consideration, calculate for two extra suppositories, i.e., for 10.

Calculation for 10 suppositories

Quantity of theobroma oil required $= 1 \times 10$

$$= 10 \text{ g} \qquad \text{(mould size = 1 g)}$$

Quantity of bismuth subgallate required $= 300 \times 10 = 3000 \text{ mg} = 3 \text{ g}$

Displacement value of bismuth subgallate $= 3$

3 g of bismuth subgallate displaces 1 g of cocoa butter

1 g of bismuth subgallate will displace 1 g of cocoa butter $= \dfrac{1}{3}$

3 g of bismuth subgallate will displace 1 g of cocoa butter $= \frac{1}{3} \times 3$

$$= 1 \text{ g}$$

Actual amount of cocoa butter required $= (1 \times 10) - 1$

(mould size = 1 g)

$$= 9 \text{ g}$$

Total weight of 10 suppositories $= 9 + 3 = 12$ g

Weight of one suppository $= \frac{12}{10} = 1.2$ g

Therefore, although made in 1 g mould, each suppository weighs 1.2 g.

2

Incompatibilities in Prescriptions

Definition

A pharmaceutical incompatibility may be defined as the result of mixing substances which are antagonistic in nature and an undesirable product is formed which may affect the safety, purpose or appearance of the preparation. These incompatibilities are of three types :

1. Physical incompatibility
2. Chemical incompatibility
3. Therapeutic incompatibilities

1. Physical incompatibility

Physical incompatibility is usually due to immiscibility, precipitate formation or liquefaction of solid materials. This may give non-uniform, unpalatable mixtures. Sometimes it becomes very difficult to measure an accurate dose from non-uniform products. Physical incompatibilities may be corrected by one or more of the following methods, i.e., order of mixing, alteration of solvents, change in the form of ingredients, alteration of volume, addition or substitution of some substances to facilitate the compounding of prescription.

Table 2.1. Examples of physical incompatibilities and their methods of correction

Reacting substances	Type of incompatibility	Method of correction
1. Oil and water	Immiscibility	Addition of emulsifying agent.
2. Indiffusible solids	Insolubility	Thickness of preparation can be increased so as to maintain the uniform distribution of preparation for a long time by adding suspending agent.

Contd.

Reacting substances	Type of incompatibility	Method of correction
3. Sulphur powder, corticosteroids	Insolubility	Addition of wetting agents like saponins.
4. Resins water	(a) Insolubility (b) Clot formation	Addition of thickening agent.
5. Menthol, camphor, thymol	Liquefaction due to the formation of eutectic mixtures.	Trituration with an absorbent like light kaolin, light magnesium carbonate.

2. Chemical incompatibility

Chemical incompatibility may be the result of chemical interactions between the ingredients of a prescription and a harmful or even dangerous product may be formed.

Generally, chemical incompatibilities result from oxidation, reduction, acid base hydrolysis or combination reaction. These reactions may be noticed by precipitation, effervescence, decomposition, colour change or by explosion and they usually occur immediately when the prescription ingredients are mixed. Sometimes the reactions proceed at a very slow rate and visible changes occur after a long time. These types of incompatibilities are known as delayed incompatibilities. Chemical incompatibilities are of two types :

(i) *Tolerated :* Interaction can be minimised by applying some suitable order of mixing but no alteration is made in the formulation of the preparation.

(ii) *Adjusted :* Interaction is prevented by addition or substitution which does not affect the medical action of the preparation.

General methods of precipitate yielding combinations

Generally, it is noticed that reaction between strong solutions proceed at a faster rate and the precipitates formed are thick and do not diffuse readily whereas the reaction between the dilute solutions proceeds at a slow rate and precipitates formed are light and diffuse readily in the solution. Hence the reacting substances should be diluted to the maximum extent before mixing them. The precipitate so formed may be diffusible or indiffusible. The methods adopted for dispensing such preparations in which diffusible or indiffusible precipitates are formed are given below :

Method A

This method is used when diffusible precipitates are formed and in those cases where the amount of precipitate formed is very small. Divide the vehicle into two equal portions. Dissolve one of the reacting substances in one portion and the other in other portion. Mix the two portions by slowly adding one portion to the other with rapid stirring.

Method B

This method is used when the indiffusible precipitates are formed and they form an appreciable portion of the mixture. Divide the vehicle into two equal portions. Dissolve one of the reacting substances in one portion. Place the other portion of the vehicle in mortar. To this add a suitable amount of compound tragacanth powder CPT (10 grains per ounce or 2 g per 100 ml of finished product) with constant trituration until a smooth mucilage is produced. Then add other reacting substances. Mix the two portions by slowing adding one portion to the other with rapid stirring.

Note : Where method A or method B has been used in dispensing the prescription, it is very important to write on the label "Shake the bottle before use.".

Table 2.2.

S. No.	Alkaloid or alkaloidal salt	Limit per oz of mixture for non-precipitation with alkaline substances	Delimiting factors	Method adopted to correct precipitation
1.	Strychnine hydrochloride	8 minims	Alcohol increases solubility	A
2.	Morphine hydrochloride	12 minims	Alcohol increases solubility	A
3.	Caffeine citrate, caffeine and sodium iodide	11 grains	Alcohol increases solubility	B
4.	Soluble quinine compounds	Very small, hence with normal doses precipitation occurs	—	B
5.	Cocaine hydrochloride	Very small, hence in normal concentration precipitation always occurs	Borax with glycerin or boric acid is compatible	Refer back to prescriber

Table 2.3. Methods of correcting chemical incompatibilities

I. Alkaloidal incompatibility

S. No.	Alkaloid or alkaloidal salt	Reacting substance	Type of precipitation or reaction	Method of correction
1.	Strychnine hydrochloride	Aromatic spirit of ammonia	Diffusible ppt.	A
2.	Ferric quinine citrate	Aromatic spirit of ammonia	Indiffusible	B
3.	All alkaloids	Tannic acid containing substances like tincture of catechu, hammelis liquid extract	Diffusible	A
4.	Quinine (alkaloidal) salts	Salicylates, benzoates	Indiffusible	B

II. Soluble iodides

S. No.	Name of iodide	Reacting substance	Type of precipitation or reaction	Method of correction
1.	Potassium iodide	Ferric chloride	$KI + FeCl_3 \rightarrow$ $I^- + KCl + FeCl_2$ Free iodide release should be prevented.	Free iodide can be prevented by adding alkali citrate/tartrate. Ferric ions are not liberated from this organic compound and due to which oxidation is prevented.

Contd.

S. No.	Name of iodide	Reacting substance	Type of precipitation or reaction	Method of correction
2.	Syrup of ferric iodide	Potassium chlorate	$KClO_3 + 3FeI_3 \rightarrow 3FeOI + 3I_2 + KCl$ This mixture is clear when prepared but deposits of crystals of iodine are formed upon standing for some time.	Hence two reacting substances should be dispensed separately.
3.	Potassium iodide	Quinine sulphate and dilute sulphuric acid	The mixture is clear at first but after 3 days it may deposit green crystals. The reaction which takes place is 'herapath reaction' for quinine and herapathite (iodosulphate of quinine) is formed $(C_{20}H_{24}O_2N_2)_4 \cdot 3H_2SO_4 \cdot 2HI \cdot 2I_2 \cdot 6H_2O$	Supply should be given for 3 days or the mixture should be divided sending the KI in one bottle and the other ingredient in other bottle and labelled with the direction "Mix both the ingredients while administration of the dose.".

III. Incompatibility of soluble salicylate and benzoates

S. No.	Name of salicylate/ benzoate	Reacting substance	Type of precipitation or reaction	Method of correction
1.	Sodium salicylate	Quinine sulphate + dil. H_2SO_4	Tolerated incompatibility. H_2SO_4 is included to dissolve quinine sulphate but at the same time, H_2SO_4 reacts with sodium salicylate and decomposes to form indiffusible ppt. of salicylic acid.	Method B

Contd.

S. No.	Name of salicylate/ benzoate	Reacting substance	Type of precipitation or reaction	Method of correction
2.	Sodium salicylate	Syrup of lemon (20 ml)	Adjusted incompatibility. Lemon syrup contains citric acid and will liberate salicylic acid from sodium salicylate.	Lemon syrup is added as a flavouring agent and hence it may be replaced by large volume of syrup (19 ml) and small volume of tr. (1.2 ml) of lemon without altering the therapeutic action of mixture.
3.	Sodium salicylate gr x	Caffeine citrate gr xv	Adjusted incompatibility. Caffeine citrate is a mixture of equal weights of caffeine and citric acid which forms salicylic acid from sodium salicylate.	With sodium salicylate, caffeine forms a very soluble compound, so that when caffeine citrate is prescribed with salicylate, as much as half of caffeine should be substituted and the mixture will be quite clear. Therefore substitute 5 gr of caffeine in place of caffeine citrate.
4.	Sodium salicylate	Ferric chloride	Indiffusible ppt. of ferric salicylate is formed.	Method B
5.	Sodium salicylate or sodium benzoate	Sodium bicarbonate + ferric chloride	Ferric salicylate is formed which is soluble in $KHCO_3/NaHCO_3$. Hence a clear mixture is obtained.	Ferric salts + sodium salicylate. Ferric salicylate indiffusible ppt. Method B for correction. Ferric salts + sodium benzoate. Ferric benzoate diffusible ppt. Method A for correction.

Contd.

IV. Incompatibility causing evolution of CO_2

S. No.	Name of bicarbonate/ carbonate	Reacting substance	Type of precipitation or reaction	Method for correction
1.	Sodium bicarbonate	Borax + glycerin	In the presence of glycerin borax decomposes to form sodium metaborate and boric acid. 1. $Na_2B_4O_7 + 3H_2O \rightarrow Na_2B_2O_4 + 3H_3BO_3$ 2. Boric acid reacts with glycerin to form a monobasic glyceryl boric acid. $2 (CH_2OH)_2CHOH + 3H_3BO_3 \rightarrow (C_3H_5)_2 (HBO_3)_3 + 6H_2O$ 3. Glyceryl boric acid reacts with bicarbonates liberating CO_2 but boric acid does not liberate CO_2 from $NaHCO_3$.	When these three substance are to be dispensed they should be mixed with water in an open vessel until effervescence ceases.
2.	Sodium bicarbonate	Bismuth subnitrate	$2BiONO_3 + 2NaHCO_3 \rightarrow (BiO_2) CO_3 + NaNO_3 + CO_2 + H_2O$ Bismuth carbonate (diffusible) is precipitated.	Method A

V. Miscellaneous

(i) Oxidation-reduction reactions

Rx

Mercurous chloride	gr	xv
Potassium bromide	gr	xxv
Sucrose	gr	xx

M. ft. Pulvis mitte tales 12.

The incompatibility of this prescription is moisture. In this, mercurous chloride reacts with potassium bromide to form mercuric bromide (reduction of mercurous chloride) and free mercury. Therefore the prescription should never be dispensed.

(ii) *Hydrolysis*

  (a) *Rx*

Sodium salicylate	8.0 g
Phenobarbital sodium	5.4 g
Vitamin B complex elixir	180 ml

The alkalinity of salts causes decomposition by hydrolysis of the vitamin B and precipitation of salicylic acid. To overcome this problem, salts should be dispensed separately.

  (b) *Rx*

Penicillin G sodium	1,000,000 IU
Syrup of cherry q.s.	30 ml

     M. ft. Solutio mitte 60 ml.

Penicillin salt gets hydrolysed in acidic media and precipitate of free acid of penicillin is formed. This can be reduced by using a neutral vehicle.

  (c) *Rx*

Potassium chlorate	0.5 g
Tannic acid	0.2 g
Sucrose	0.2 g

     M. ft. Pulvis send 20 g.

As this is an explosive combination so ingredients can be compounded with minimum rubbing or each ingredient can be powdered individually and dispensed separately with a special direction on the label.

3. Therapeutic incompatibility

Therapeutic incompatibility may be the result of prescribing certain drugs to the patient with the intention to produce a specific degree of action but the nature or the intensity of action produced is different from that intended by the prescriber. It may be due to the following reasons :

  (i) Overdose

 (ii) Synergism

(iii) Antagonism

(iv) Contraindication

(i) Overdose

This incompatibility is present when the dose of a drug in a prescription is excessive. Sometimes the overdosage is intentional. For example, aspirin may be prescribed in large doses for the relief of rheumatoid arthiritis.

However when potent drugs like atropine are prescribed in overdose, it is the duty of the pharmacist to contact the prescriber and get it corrected, otherwise the dispensing of such prescription may lead to fatal consequences.

(ii) Synergism

When two drugs are prescribed together they tend to increase the activity of each other. This is known as synergism. Synergism is usually intentional because the prescriber has prescribed the drugs together wishing to secure the increased activity. A combination of aspirin and paracetamol increases analgesic activity. A combination of penicillin and streptomycin increases antibacterial activity. Since this synergism is intentional therefore there is no objection to it.

However when two depressants are prescribed together, it may lead to disastrous consequences. The prescriber should be contacted immediately for the prescription.

(iii) Antagonism

When two drugs having opposing pharmacological effects are prescribed together, this incompatibility is present. However, this may be intentional, e.g., a CNS stimulant may be prescribed to counteract an excessive sedative effect of phenobarbitone in epilepsy. Similarly a sedative may be prescribed along with ephedrine in asthma to reduce the side effect of CNS stimulation by ephedrine.

However, there may be instances when the prescriber prescribes two drugs together without being aware of the chemical interaction between them resulting in reduced absorption and in reduced efficacy. For example tetracycline cannot be prescribed together with antacids (aluminium and magnesium compounds), iron preparations, and calcium salts, since complexation of these metals by the tetracycline takes place. This results in reduced absorption of tetracycline.

Rx

Tetracycline   250 mg

Make capsules, send such 20 capsules.

Direction : Every capsule should be taken with milk 8 hourly.

In this prescription the direction is wrong. Tetracycline is inactivated by calcium which is present in milk. Therefore tetracycline capsules should not be taken with milk. Hence refer the prescription back to the prescriber for change in direction.

3

Posology

Dose and Dosage of Drugs

Dose of a drug can be defined as the amount which produces required therapeutic effect in adults for which it is indicated. The normal dosage range for a drug indicates the amount of drug that may be prescribed within the framework of usual medical practice. Doses falling outside of the normal dosage range may be questioned by the pharmacist for further scrutiny and consultation with the prescriber.

The schedule of dosage or the **dosage regimen** is generally given along with the drug, e.g., some drugs are taken every 6 hourly or at bed time or after meals, etc. There are few terms which are used to describe schedule of dosage, e.g., Digoxin requires **initial dose** to attain the desired concentration of the drug in the blood. Then subsequent doses are administered to maintain that level through **maintenance dose**. Similarly **prophylactic dose** is the amount which is administered for prevention of disease. **Therapeutic dose** is given after exposure to illness to cure the patient.

Principles governing the dosage schedule generally depend upon pharmacokinetic properties, pharmacodynamic properties, and the characteristics of the disease. Because dosage regimen varies with patient and illness, one must not forget the following points before tailoring a dosage schedule for a patient :

1. Look up the dosage regimens recommended in official books.

2. Check up for its dose related toxicity. If the drug has low therapeutic ratio, precautions should be taken not to give **overdose**.

3. Dose-response curve for the patient must be considered.

4. Consider the characteristics of the patient, e.g., age, weight, sex, renal and hepatic functions, etc.

5. Drug interactions.

6. Consider whether initial/loading dose is required or not.

Factors Influencing Dose

There are number of factors which affect the dose of a drug. These are described as follows :

  (i)   Age
 (ii)   Sex
(iii)   Route, method and time of drug administration
(iv)   Body weight
 (v)   Environment
(vi)   Genetic factors
(vii)   Time of administration
(viii) Route of administration
(ix)   Emotional factors
 (x)   Metabolic disturbances ·
(xi)   Presence of disease
(xii)   Cumulation
(xiii) Additive effect
(xiv)   Synergism
(xv)   Antagonism

(i) Age

Children and old persons require lesser amount of drug. In neonates membrane permeability and blood brain barrier permeability is greater as compared to adults. Therefore, for infant's and children's doses certain rules have to be followed like Young's rule, Clark's rule, Dilling's rule, etc.

(ii) Sex

Females require 0.85 of the male dose because of their lesser weight and they are more receptive to drugs. Less dose is given to female during :

  (a) Menstruation
  (b) Pregnancy
  (c) Lactation

(iii) Route, method and time of administration

The method of drug administration counts a lot. Injections are quickly and more completely absorbed as against a tablet or capsule. Similarly drugs are better and rapidly absorbed in an empty stomach.

(iv) **Body weight**

While calculating a dose, weight of the person should be considered, e.g., the average dose is mentioned either in terms of mg per kg body weight or as the total single dose for an adult weighing between 50-100 kg.

(v) **Environment**

The amount of barbiturates required during daytime to produce sleep is much higher than the dose required at night.

(vi) **Genetic factors**

The science of pharmacogenetics is concerned with variations due to genetic factors. It has been found that patients with genetic metabolic disorders rarely show a disturbance in the metabolism of drugs because the microsomal enzymes (involved in metabolism) do not participate in the intermediary metabolism.

   (i) Acetylation of drugs : The rate of acetylation of INH, procainamide, sulfonamides is controlled by an autosomal recessive gene and the dosage of these drugs depends upon the acetylator status of individuals.
   (ii) Glucose-6-phosphate dehydrogenase : Primaquine causes haemolysis in individuals having deficiency of glucose-6-phosphate dehydrogenase.

(vii) **Time of administration**

Drugs which are taken after meals cause less gastric irritation, nausea and vomitting. Generally food content slows down the rate and extent of absorption, e.g., tetracyclines are contra-indicated with milk (calcium salts).

(viii) **Route of administration**

I.V. route requires less dose than oral route. The onset of drug action is much quicker with I.V. route.

(ix) **Emotional factors**

When the drug is meant for psychosomatic disorders, generally placebos (inert dosage form) are given. Placebos are known to produce therapeutic benefit in conditions like angina pectoris, and bronchial asthma.

(x) Metabolic disturbances

Changes in electrolyte balance, body temperature, etc., may modify the effects of drugs, e.g., salicylates reduce body temperature only in fever while they have no antipyretic effect in normal conditions.

(xi) Presence of disease

Drugs like barbiturates and chlorpromazine may produce unusually prolonged effect in cirrhotic patients.

(xii) Cumulation

When the drug is excreted slowly, its continuous administration may produce toxicity. To avoid cumulation one must know about its rate of elimination and the form in which it should be administered. One should check liver and kidney function.

(xiii) Additive effect

When two or more drugs are administered together, pharmacological action is equivalent to the summation of their individual pharmacological action.

(xiv) Synergism

The word synergism is derived from Greek words. It indicates a pharmacologic cooperation. In this when two or more drugs are given together, one drug facilitates the action of other.

(xv) Antagonism

When two drugs are given together and they oppose actions of each other, the pharmacological action is called antagonism. It is of following types :

   (i) Chemical antagonism

  (ii) Competitive or reversible antagonism

 (iii) Non-competitive antagonism

CALCULATION OF DOSES FOR CHILDREN

The following formulas are useful :

1. Young's formula

$$\frac{\text{Age in years} \times \text{Adult dose}}{\text{Age} + 12} = \text{Dose for the child}$$

The formula is used for calculating the doses for children under 12 years of age.

2. Dilling's formula

$$\frac{\text{Age in years} \times \text{Adult dose}}{20} = \text{Dose for the child}$$

This formula is used for calculating the dose for children between 4 to 20 years of age.

3. Cowling's formula

$$\frac{\text{Age in years} + 1}{24} \times \text{Adult dose} = \text{Dose for the child}$$

4. Fried's formula

$$\frac{\text{Age in months}}{150} \times \text{Adult dose} = \text{Dose for the child}$$

5. Bastedo's formula

$$\frac{\text{Age in years} + 3}{30} \times \text{Adult dose} = \text{Dose for the child}$$

6. Clark's formula

$$\frac{\text{Weight in pounds}}{150} \times \text{Adult dose} = \text{Dose for the child}$$

7. Goubin's formula

Under 1 year	=	1/12 of the adult dose
From 1-2 years	=	1/8 of the adult dose
From 2-3 years	=	1/6 of the adult dose
From 3-4 years	=	1/4 of the adult dose
From 4-7 years	=	1/3 of the adult dose
From 7-14 years	=	1/2 of the adult dose
From 14-20 years	=	2/3 of the adult dose
From 21-60 years	=	Full adult dose
From 60-70 years	=	4/5 of the adult dose
From 70-80 years	=	3/4 of the adult dose
From 80-90 years	=	2/3 of the adult dose
Over 90 years	=	1/2 of the adult dose

8. Formula based on body surface

$$\log S = 0.425 \log w + 0.725 \log h + 1.8564$$

where s = surface area

w = weight in kg
h = height in cm.

The surface area can be calculated from the monograms constructed using the above formula.

Veterinary Dosage

As the pharmacist is responsible for correct dosage in any type of prescription, therefore he must study posology which pertains to animal medications. Veterinary doses vary according to the type of animal, large or small. These dosages are usually stated on a unit per pound basis; however, some are given as average dosages for the various species.

In veterinary medicines, 'history taking' is the most important aspect for clinical examination because animals are unable to describe their symptoms and signs. They vary widely in their reaction to handling and examination, e.g., variations from normal physiological functions such as intake of food or drink, milk production, growth, respiration, defecation, urination, sweating, posture, activity, voice and odour should be noted in all cases.

Veterinary dosage for a 40 lb. adult dog is approximately the same as for a 150 lb. mature man. If we assign the dose for an adult dog as (1), values for other animals can be compared as follows : cats (0.5), swine (2), sheep and goats (3), horses (16) and cattle (24). Generally the dose for animals from birth up to a few weeks old is approximately 1/20 of adult dose. For half-grown animals, the dose is about 1/3 of the adult dose.

4
Powders

Definition

Powders are the solid dosage of medicament which are meant for internal and external use and are available in crystalline or amorphous form.

Advantages

(i) They are the easiest to prescribe, compound and administer because most of the drugs are available in powder forms.
(ii) They are easier to carry than liquids.
(iii) Stability is much better when compared to other dosage forms.
(iv) Chances of incompatibility are less.
(v) They have got more surface area, so rapid dissolution occurs which increases the blood concentration in a shorter time and thereby action is produced in a lesser time.
(vi) Children and infants cannot swallow tablets and capsules and under such circumstances drugs can be administered in powder form making them palatable by mixing with milk, fruit juice or honey.
(vii) They are more economical because they do not require any special technique or machinery for their preparation.

Disadvantages

(i) Volatile, hygroscopic, oxidizing and deliquescent drugs create problems in dispensing.
(ii) Bitter, nauseous and corrosive drugs cannot be dispensed in powder form.

Classification of Powders

1. Divided powders
2. Bulk powders
3. Granules or effervescent granules
4. Special powders
5. Dental powders
6. Tablet triturates
7. Cachets.

1. Divided powders

They are of two types :
- (i) Simple powders
- (ii) Compound powders.

(i) *Simple powders*

A simple powder contains only one ingredient either in crystalline or amorphous form. When the powder is in the crystalline form, then it should be reduced to fine powder, weighed and wrapped as individual doses.

(ii) *Compound powders*

Compound powder contains two or more than two substances which are mixed together and then divided into individual doses.

Method of preparation

1. Separately powder a slight excess of each crystalline substance.
2. Weigh out the required amount of each powder and diluent, i.e., lactose, if necessary.
3. Triturate all the ingredients in ascending order of their weights thoroughly so that a homogenous powder is formed.
4. Weigh out the required number of powders and wrap them in the papers.
5. If the powder is of volatile nature or hygroscopic substance, then double wrapping should be done in which the inner paper should be of wax paper to prevent volatilization and absorption of moisture.

2. Bulk powders

Powders supplied in bulk quantities are applied by the patient according to his need. They are preferably supplied in perforated or sifter type containers.

(i) *Dusting powders*

(a) Dusting powders are meant for external application to the skin for antiseptic, antipruritic, astringent, absorbent, protective and antiperspirant purposes.

(b) Dusting powders should flow easily and should be able to protect the skin from irritation caused by friction, moisture or chemical irritants. These powders must be in a very fine state of subdivision for their effectiveness and to minimise local irritation. Therefore they should be passed through a sieve No. 120.

(c) Dusting powders are of two types :

1. *Medical :* These powders are used mainly for superficial skin conditions and are not intended for open wounds or areas of broken skin, so sterility is not essential. However, they must be free from pathogens. Some mineral ingredients (e.g., light kaolin and talc) may be contaminated with spores of tetanus or gas gangrene. Therefore, they should be sterilised for using in the formulation.

2. *Surgical :* These powders are used in body cavities and on major wounds. Therefore, they must be sterilised. They often contain an antibacterial agent and the diluent which may be sterilisable maize starch, also known as absorbable dusting powder.

(d) Dusting powders are dispensed in sifter top containers or pressure aerosols. The pressure aerosol containers are costlier than other containers but can protect the powder from atmospheric condition and help in the easy application of the preparations. They can also be applied with powder puff or a soft brush or a sterilised gauze pad but care must be taken to avoid mechanical irritation to the skin surface.

(e) As these powders are in a very fine state of subdivision they may cause pulmonary inflammation of lungs in infants and absorption of boric acid through the broken skin. So proper care must be taken while handling these preparations.

(ii) *Insufflations*

Insufflations are the fine powders which are used to produce :

   (i) a local effect, as in the treatment of ear, nose and throat infection with antibiotics;

   (ii) a systemic effect, from a drug which gets destroyed in the gut.

These powders are applied with the help of an apparatus known as **insufflator**. This divides the powder into a stream of finely divided particles to the site of application. The major difficulty in using this apparatus is that :

   (i) it is difficult to obtain a measured quantity of drug to get a uniform dose;

   (ii) it has a tendency to get blocked when the powders used are wet or the apparatus itself is wet.

The introduction of newer pressure aerosols have eliminated these difficulties. The diluents normally used for insufflations are lactose and for preparations applied to open wounds and raw surfaces, sterilisable maize starch.

(iii) *Snuffs*

These are the finely divided solid dosage form of medicament which are inhaled into the nostrils for their antiseptic, decongestion or bronchodilator action.

3. Effervescent granules

Effervescent granules are the specially prepared solid dosage form of the medicament, meant for internal use. They usually contain a soluble medicinal agent mixed with citric acid, tartaric acid and sodium bicarbonate. Before administration they are suspended, dissolved in water or are mixed with soft drinks. On mixing with water, carbon dioxide is released as a result of acid-base reaction. This mixture should be taken while effervescing.

Formula for effervescent granules

Effervescent granules consist of the following ingredients :

1. **Sodium bicarbonate.** It reacts with the acids when the preparation is added to water. The evolved carbon dioxide produces effervescence.

2. **Citric and tartaric acids.** The quantity of these acids is slightly more than is necessary to neutralise the sodium bicarbonate because effervescent preparations are more palatable if slightly acid. The relative proportion of these two acids is based upon the quantity of water needed to make the material coherent. Tartaric acid is anhydrous, but citric acid has one molecule of water of crystallisation equal to 8.75% of its weight. On heating the mixture of the acids and bicarbonates, water is liberated and provides the moist condition to produce coherent mass.

Chemical reaction

$$3NaHCO_3 + C_6H_8O_7 \rightarrow C_6H_5Na_3O_7 + 3CO_2 + 3H_2O$$
$$\text{Citric acid} \qquad \text{Sodium citrate}$$

$$2NaHCO_3 + C_4H_6O_6 \rightarrow C_4H_4Na_2O_6 + 2CO_2 + 2H_2O$$
$$\text{Tartaric acid} \qquad \text{Sodium tartrate}$$

The water from these two sources (i.e., water of crystallization of citric acid and that formed by interaction between the acids and bicarbonate) makes the material coherent.

Citric acid

Citric acid serves two purposes : (i) it provides most of the moisture needed for granulation; (ii) it neutralises part of the bicarbonate.

Tartaric acid

The amount of tartaric acid is slightly more than that required to neutralise the sodium bicarbonate, the excess giving a pleasant acid flavour to the preparation.

Medicament

The medicament used in an effervescent preparation must be free from any water of crystallization which is liberated at or below 100°C (temperature of granulation).

Sweetening agent

Sucrose or more often saccharin may be added.

Method of preparation

There are two methods of preparation of effervescent granules :

    (i) Heat method

    (ii) Wet method

(i) *Heat method*

1. A large porcelain or stainless steel evaporating dish is placed over a water bath, with as much of the dish as possible exposed to the water or steam and the water is heated to boiling point. The dish should be hot enough so that when powders are added to it, it should provide sufficient water needed for granulation which will be liberated by citric acid on heating.
2. All the powdered ingredients are passed through sieve No. 60, weighed and mixed.
3. Then they are placed in the dish already warmed on water bath.
4. The mass is pressed with spatula until the mixture forms a coherent damp mass.
5. The damp mass is then passed through sieve to prepare granules.
6. Granules are then dried by keeping them in an oven at a temperature not exceeding 60°C.
7. Dried granules are packed in dry, wide-mouth and air-tight containers.

(ii) *Wet method*

1. Mixed ingredients are moistened with the help of some suitable vehicle (for which alcohol is most suitable) with continuous stirring until a coherent mass is formed.
2. This coherent mass is then passed through a sieve to prepare granules.
3. These granules are then dried at a temperature not exceeding 60°C.
4. Dried granules are again passed through sieve to break the lumps which may have been formed during drying.
5. Dried granules are packed in dry, wide-mouth and air-tight containers.

4. Special powders

1. Eutectic mixtures
2. Hygroscopic and deliquescent powders
3. Efflorescent powders
4. Liquids
5. Explosive substances
6. Potent drugs
7. Granular powders
8. Vegetable powders.

1. *Eutectic mixtures*

Some of the drugs when mixed together tend to liquefy due to the formation of new compound. These mixtures have a melting point below room temperature. Such mixtures are called eutectic mixtures. Substances which on mixing liquefy are menthol, thymol, camphor, phenol, salol, chloral hydrate, aminopyrine, aspirin, phenacetin.

These type of mixtures can be dispensed by different methods :

(i) By adding an inert absorbent like magnesium carbonate, light magnesium oxide, kaolin, starch, lactose.
(ii) They can be dispensed in separate sets of powders and labelled with suitable direction.

2. *Hygroscopic and deliquescent powders*

Substances which absorb moisture from the atmosphere are called hygroscopic and if the content of water absorbed is high which makes the material liquid it is called a deliquescent solid, e.g., hyoscine hydrobromide, phenobarbitone sodium, potassium citrate, pepsin, ammonium chloride, ammonium bromide, ammonium iodide, citric acid, tartaric acid, sodium bromide and sodium iodide. Several precautions are to be taken to dispense such powders :

(i) Supply the drug in granular form to provide the minimum exposure to atmosphere.

(ii) Double wrapping should be done in which waxed paper is used for inner lining. In highly humid climate one may use aluminium foil or plastic packets for preventing the access of air.

3. *Efflorescent powders*

Crystalline substances which liberate water of crystallization due to change in humidity are called efflorescent substances. The only remedy to avoid this process is to use anhydrous salt of the corresponding substance. However, allowance should be made for water of crystallization when calculations are done. Examples : caffeine, cocaine, codeine phosphate, quinine bisulfate, alum, atropine sulphate, sodium acetate, sodium carbonate, sodium phosphate.

4. *Liquids*

When the amount of liquid is small, it may be triturated with an equal quantity of powder, then the other ingredients should be added in small amounts with continuous trituration. If the quantities of liquids are large, an absorbent should be added. For tinctures and liquid extracts, they should be evaporated to the consistency of a syrup. Add lactose or any other suitable diluent and continue evaporation to dryness. Then add other ingredients. Addition of diluent prevents the formation of sticky mass on evaporation.

5. *Explosive substances*

When some oxidising and reducing substance is triturated in a mortar, there are chances of explosion. Though such combinations are rare, but if it has to be dispensed then powder each ingredient and dispense them separately with a special direction for its use.

6. *Potent drug*

Drugs having a maximum dose of less than one grain and poisonous substances should be regarded as potent substances. As the dose is very less, so we have to prepare triturations. In this method, the drug is reduced to fine powder and to this an equal amount of diluent is mixed well by thorough trituration in a mortar. To this is added the rest of the diluent in successive portions with thorough trituration each time until whole of the diluent has been added. It should be kept in mind that whole of the diluent should not be added to the drug otherwise the potent drug will not be mixed uniformly and will result in uneven distribution of drug in divided powders.

7. Granular powders

Some of the antibiotics (e.g., phenoxy methyl penicillin potassium) are unstable in solution or suspension, therefore they are formulated by manufacturers as dry granules containing the medicaments and various additives such as buffering, preservative, colouring, flavouring, dispersing and suspending agents. They are packed in bottles large enough to hold the water that is added when a prescription is received.

8. Vegetable powders

These powders contain volatile oils which should not be subjected to heavy grinding in a mortar. They must be powdered lightly in a mortar to prevent the loss of volatile oil present in them. As these powders contain volatile substances they must be double wrapped with a inner wrapping of a waxed paper.

5. Dental powders

These powders are meant for cleaning the teeth. A dental powder contains detergents, abrasives, antiseptics, colouring and flavouring agents incorporated in a suitable base. Generally the base is calcium carbonate. The detergent is in the form of soap. A mild degree of abrasion may be obtained by using different calcium salts like finely precipitated calcium carbonate, dibasic calcium phosphate, calcium sulphate, magnesium carbonate. Essential oils are added to provide flavours and freshness to the mouth as well as antiseptic action. Essential oils, if present in smaller quantity, are easily absorbed by calcium carbonate. This makes uniform distribution of oil difficult. Best results are obtained if the oil is triturated in the solid, taking considerable care to distribute it uniformly.

6. Tablet triturates

These are the powders which are moulded in the form of a tablet. Generally potent medicaments and highly toxic drugs in small doses are used for preparing molded tablet. The tablet triturates retain their shape under normal conditions and may be swallowed as a whole or crushed into a powder. The potent medicament is mixed with a diluent like sucrose, dextrose or lactose. The mixed powder is then moistened with sufficient quantity of alcohol to get a soft mass. This soft mass is pressed into perforations of upper plate. A spatula is used to ensure that each cavity is filled. The filled cavity is then pressed down on the lower plate leaving the molded tablets on the projecting pegs. The ejected tablets are left for drying on clean surface either in a warm place or in a hot air oven.

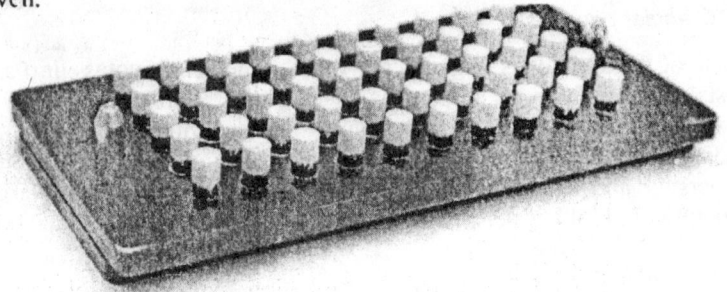

Fig. 4.1. Tablet triturate mould.

Nowadays automatic tablet triturate machines are available which can prepare 2500 tablet triturates per minute.

7. Cachets

Cachets are unit dosage form made by pouring a mixture of rice flour and water between two hot, polished revolving cylinders. Water evaporates and sheet of wafer is formed. For administration they are softened by immersion in water for few seconds and then taken with a draught of water.

Advantages

1. They are used for nauseous and disagreeable powders.
2. Large doses of drugs can be administered.
3. No complicated machinery is required.
4. They disintegrate quickly in stomach.

Disadvantages

1. More space is required because of fragile nature of shells.
2. They are less resistant to light and moisture.
3. They must be softened before swallowing.
4. They get easily damaged.

Cachets are of two types :

1. Wet seal
2. Dry seal

1. *Wet seal cachets*

These cachets require machine which consists of three metal plates joined by hinges. Each plate has two or more similar holes so that it can be used for different sizes of cachets. In wet seal cachets there are two halves, convex in shape and water is used to seal them.

Method of preparation

1. Weigh and mix the ingredients. Pass through sieve No. 250.
2. Clean the machine thoroughly and open it. Place cachets over plates.
3. Choose the correct funnel and thimble according to the size of cachet.
4. Place the funnel over the first hole and carefully tip the powder.
5. Press down gently with thimble.
6. Gently remove thimble and funnel.
7. The covering plate is turned back, the flange of the empty half of the cachet is moistened with water so that two halves of cachets can be joined by slight pressure.
8. Dry the cachets for about 15 minutes.

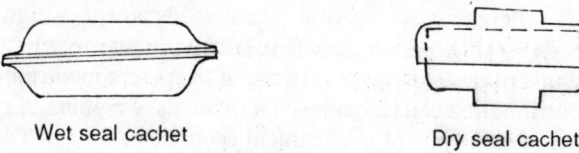

Wet seal cachet   Dry seal cachet

Fig. 4.2.

2. *Dry seal cachets*

They have shallow cylindrical base and a slightly larger, slip-over cap. One variety of dry seal cachets consists of a cylindrical dome at the centre of the top and base is generally used to fix the cachet in the machine. The other type consists of two hinged plates along with holes of same size as the stud on cachet. Plates are opened, the smaller half of the cachet is placed on the lower plate, stud fitting loosely into one of the holes. A loose plate with hole is then kept over it. Powder is poured through the hole of loose plate, which is then removed. The cap of the cachet is then pressed over forcing the cap over lower half.

Weighing technique

The powdered drug is weighed accurately with the help of a balance.

1. A watch glass or a butter paper with a suitable counterpoise is used for the placement of drug.
2. All the ingredients are weighed one after another and kept separately.
3. Emphasis should be given that the drug should not be touched with hands at any stage.
4. Weights should be removed from the box and replaced using forceps.

Minimum weighable amounts

It is generally accepted that the error in the amount of any ingredient in a dispensed preparation should not be more than 5%. It is advisable to make 100 mg or 2 grains as the minimum weighable amounts for dispensing balance.

Weighing of material below the minimal amounts

Potent substances used in small doses are mixed with diluents such as lactose, calcium phosphate, etc., so as to weigh out uniform doses accurately. For this purpose triturates are prepared by mixing definite quantities of the potent medicament with definite quantities of the diluents. For weighing 10 mg of a potent medicament, weigh 100 mg and mix with 900 mg of lactose. The resultant mixture weighs 1000 mg. 100 mg of this triturate represents 10 mg of the potent medicament. Like this further trituration can be made to facilitate the weighing of even very small doses of some potent medicament accurately.

Geometric dilution

While mixing the ingredients this method should be adopted. In this, the ingredient in the lowest quantity, say 100 mg, is taken first in the mortar. It is mixed with an equal quantity of any other ingredient or the diluent. The total weight of mixture is 200 mg. So 200 mg of the diluent is now added to the mortar. Next 400 mg are added and so on till all the ingredients are added. This method ensures complete and uniform mixing of all ingredients and accurate doses of the medicament can be easily weighed out.

Proper usage and care of dispensing balance

In using a prescription balance neither the weights nor the substance that is to be weighed should be placed on the pans when the beam is oscillating. The desired weight should be placed upon the R.H.S. pan and substance to be weighed should be placed upon the opposite pan. The beam should be released by means of the lever and if the substance is in excess, the beam should be locked. Small portion is removed with the help of a spatula and the beam is again released. The oscillations are observed. This procedure should be repeated until the correct amount is obtained. In case of a deficiency of the substance to be weighed the reverse procedure is followed until the correct amount is obtained.

Substances which react with metals like iodine, corrosive sublimates, etc., should not be weighed directly upon pans, but ,with the help of glazed paper. Care should be taken to balance the papers before weighing the substance. Polishing powders are sometimes used for cleaning purpose.

5

Monophasic Liquid Dosage Form

The use of liquid oral dosage form is justified on the basis of ease of administration and rapid absorption to those individuals who cannot swallow solid dosage form. Since drugs are absorbed in their dissolved state more rapidly, their absorption rate decreases in the following order:

aqueous solution > aqueous suspension > tablet or capsule

Liquid oral dosage forms can be classified as:

(i) Monophasic liquid dosage form:

    (a) Liquids for internal administration — mixtures, syrups and elixirs.

    (b) Liquids meant for external administration or used on mucous membrane — gargles, mouth washes, throat paints, douches, ear drops, liniment, lotions.

(ii) Biphasic liquid dosage form:

    (a) Suspensions

    (b) Emulsions

Monophasic Liquid Dosage Form

The term 'monophasic liquid dosage form' refers to liquid preparation in which there is only one phase, e.g., solutions. A solution is a clear, homogenous mixture that is prepared by dissolving a solid, liquid or gas in another liquid. The component of solution present in large amount is known as solvent and the component present in lesser amount is known as solute.

Additives

(i) Vehicle

A vehicle is a medium in which the ingredients of a formulation are dissolved, suspended or dispersed for their easy administration and rapid pharmacological action. The vehicles which are most commonly used are:

(a) *Water*

(a) Water is one of the most widely used vehicles for pharmaceutical users. Its main advantage is that many drugs are water soluble and it is neutral in nature. Its availability is abundant and is not expensive.

(b) It can be made free from impurities and must be boiled and cooled before using it.

(b) *Aromatic waters*

They are used for their flavours and they contain mild preservative actions. Examples : chloroform water, camphor water, cinnamon water.

(c) *Infusions*

They have definite therapeutic actions. Examples : orange peel infusion, infusion of clove.

(d) *Alcohol*

(i) Provides antimicrobial properties.

(ii) Mixtures of alcohol and water are used in any preparation to increase the solubility (hydroalcoholic mixture).

(e) *Glycerin*

It is a polyhydric alcohol of good viscosity and is mostly used in throat paints because of its viscous nature as it remains in contact with mucous membrane of the throat for a longer time. It has got a sweet taste.

(ii) **Stabilizers**

Stabilizers are the substances which ensures the physical and chemical stability of the drugs. The most important stabilisers are :

(a) Antioxidants

(b) Preservatives

(a) *Antioxidants*

Antioxidants provide protection to the drug from oxygen by combining with themselves. They have great affinity for oxygen. An antioxidant should be non-irritant, non-toxic, colourless, thermostable, and compatible. Examples : sodium bisulphite, sodium metabisulphite, sodium thiosulphate, ascorbic acid, propyl gallates, (BHT) butylated hydroxy toluene, (BHA) butylated hydroxy anisole.

(b) *Preservatives*

Preservatives are added to pharmaceutical preparations to prevent the growth of microorganism in the preparations.

Liquid dosage forms generally contain water which is a good medium for multiplication of bacteria and moulds. Therefore preservatives are added to all formulations which are stored for long time. A preservative should be non-toxic, non-irritant, effective over wide range of micro-organism. The commonly used preservatives are benzoic acid, salicylic acid, phenol, benzalkonium chloride, alcohol, methyl paraben, propyl paraben.

(iii) Colouring agents

These agents are added to the formulation so as to give a good and colourful appearance to increase the acceptability of the preparation. Colours may be obtained from :

  (i) plants, e.g., chlorophyll, indigo, saffron;

  (ii) minerals, e.g., red ferric oxide, yellow ferric oxide;

  (iii) animals, e.g., cochineal.

Nowadays synthetic colours are available, e.g., nitro dyes, azo dyes, caramel or burnt sugar. An artificial colour is used to produce brown colour in cough syrups and other oral liquid preparations.

(iv) Flavouring agents

These agents are added to improve pharmaceutical preparation with a disagreeable or nauseating odour and make them more agreeable and acceptable to the patient. These preparations are generally flavoured with fruity and spicy flavours. Flavours from natural sources include banana, cardamom, cinnamon, peppermint, clove oil, lemon, orange, rose, jasmine, menthol, etc. Mannitol, chloroform water are also widely used as flavouring agents. Synthetic flavours include esters, aldehydes and alcohols. They should be stable, compatible, and of uniform composition.

Liquid Preparations for Internal Administration

Liquid preparations for internal use can be classed into three categories of preparations, namely :

  1. Mixtures

  2. Concentrated syrups

  3. Elixirs

1. Mixtures

Mixture is a liquid medicine for internal use of which several doses are contained in one bottle.

Classification of mixtures

  (i) Simple mixture containing soluble substances.
 (ii) Mixtures containing diffusible solids.
(iii) Mixtures containing indiffusible solids.
 (iv) Mixtures containing precipitates forming liquids.
  (v) Mixtures containing slightly soluble liquids.

(i) Simple mixtures containing soluble substance

These include substances which are readily soluble in water, e.g., NH_4Cl, NH_4HCO_3, $CaCl_2$, citric acid, KBr, $KHCO_3$, NaCl, Na_2CO_3, $ZnSO_4$.

It further includes substances which require powdering before dissolution due to their poor aqueous solubility, e.g., alum, borax, boric acid, caffeine citrate, potassium nitrate.

Method of preparation

1. Dissolve the solid ingredient in 3/4th of the vehicle.
2. Examine the solution by holding it against the light. If foreign particles are visible pass the solution through cotton wool.
3. Add any liquid ingredient. After measuring, rinse the vessel used with a little of aqueous vehicle and add the contents to the measuring device.
4. Add more of vehicle to produce required volume in a graduated measuring cylinder.
5. Transfer the mixture into the bottle. Finally thoroughly clean the bottle to remove finger marks. Attach the label and wrap the bottle.

(ii) Mixtures containing diffusible solids

These solids do not dissolve in water but may be mixed upon shaking and give uniform distribution of dose. These include substances mentioned below :

Bismuth carbonate, chalk powder, bismuth subnitrate, compound kaolin powder, light kaolin, $MgCO_3$ (heavy or light), MgO (heavy or light) quinine sulphate, etc.

Substances, if prescribed in a quantity greater than required, will dissolve rapidly, e.g., borax, boric acid, caffeine citrate, potassium chloride, etc.

Method of preparation

1. Finely powder the substance, add any soluble substance if present. Mix them. Measure about 3/4th of the vehicle. Add a portion of it to the mortar. Triturate to form a smooth cream. Then add remaining vehicle.

2. Observe the contents for foreign particles if present, pass the contents through muslin cloth. Rinse the mortar with little of vehicle.

3. Add any liquid ingredient, mix and transfer the mixture into measuring cylinder.

4. Add more of vehicle to produce the required volume.

5. Transfer the mixture into bottle. Then thoroughly clean the bottle to remove finger marks. Attach the label with a direction "Shake the bottle well before use.". Wrap the bottle.

(iii) *Mixture containing indiffusible solids*

Indiffusible solids are those solids which are not soluble in water and do not remain uniformly distributed in the vehicle for sufficiently long time. Therefore, to suspend the drug suspending agents are added. Indiffusible solids include acetyl salicylic acid, barbitone, benzoic acid, calomel, phenacetin, phenobarbitone, quinidine sulphate, quinine salicylate, sulfadimidine, etc.

Suspending agents which are used for indiffusible solids are :

(i) *Compound tragacanth powder :* Quantity of compound tragacanth powder is 10 grains/ounce of the mixture or 2 g/100 ml of the mixture.

Compound tragacanth powder is used when the vehicle is other than water or chloroform water.

(ii) *Tragacanth mucilage :* It is used when the vehicle is water or chloroform water. Quantity of tragacanth mucilage used is 1/4th of the volume of the mixture.

Method of preparation using compound tragacanth powder

1. Finely powder the indiffusible solid, diffusible solid and soluble substance in a mortar. To this add compound powder of tragacanth. Mix them uniformly. Measure about 3/4th of the vehicle. Triturate the powder with a portion of it until a smooth cream is formed. Then add remainder of vehicle.

2. Examine the contents of the preparation, if any foreign particle is visible, pass the contents through muslin cloth. Rinse the mortar with little of vehicle.

3. Add any liquid ingredient if present and transfer the mixture into measuring cylinder.

4. Add more of the vehicle to produce required volume in a graduated measuring cylinder.

5. Transfer the mixture into the bottle. Then thoroughly clean the bottle. Attach the label with a direction "Shake the bottle well before use.". Wrap and dispense the preparation.

Method of preparation using tragacanth mucilage

1. Finely powder the indiffusible substance in a mortar and add any soluble or diffusible solids. Mix them uniformly. Triturate the material with tragacanth mucilage (1/4th of the volume) to form a smooth cream. Then gradually dilute with 1/2 of the vehicle. The product will measure about 3/4th of the vehicle.

   Steps 2, 3, 4 and 5 are the same as described above in compound tragacanth powder method.

(iv) *Mixture containing precipitate forming liquids*

When some resinous substances are mixed with water, resin is precipitated and may adhere to the side of bottle which do not diffuse upon shaking. Therefore compound tragacanth powder or tragacanth mucilage are used. Examples are ammoniated solution of quinine, compound tincture of benzoin, etc.

Method of preparation using compound tragacanth powder

1. Finely powder the indiffusible solid and diffusible solids in the mortar. Measure 3/4th of the vehicle and to this add a portion of it and triturate to form a smooth cream. Add remainder of vehicle. Measure precipitate forming liquids in a dry container and add this into the centre of cream. Add any soluble substance to it if present. Shake it well until dissolved.

   Steps 2 to 5 are same as in case of indiffusible mixture.

Method of preparation using tragacanth mucilage

1. Mix tragacanth mucilage with an equal volume of aqueous vehicle. Measure precipitate forming liquids in a dry vessel and add slowly into the centre of mortar with constant stirring. Dissolve any solid in about 1/4th of the vehicle and mix them thoroughly.

   Steps 2 to 5 are same as mentioned in indiffusible mixture.

2. Concentrated syrups

Syrups are concentrated aqueous preparations of a sugar or sugar substitute with or without added flavouring agent and medicinal substances. Syrups containing flavouring agent but not medicinal substances are called non-medicated or flavoured vehicles. These syrups serve as pleasant tasting vehicles for medicinal substance to be added later on. When a syrup contains a therapeutic or medicinal agent then the preparation is a medicated syrup. Syrups provide a pleasant means of administering a liquid form of a disagreeable tasting drug.

Syrups are also made now by using sorbitol which is a hexahydric alcohol made by the reduction of dextrose. It is available as a white solid and is used in the form of 70% solution. Polyhydric alcohols are added in small amounts for inhibiting crystallization of sucrose.

For the manufacture of syrups, 65% weight by weight (w/w) concentration is considered. Dilute solution of sucrose (less than 65% w/w) may support mould and bacterial growth and a saturated solution of sucrose may lead to crystallization. Syrups on the other hand are devoid of both the handicaps and limitations. It is advisable to prepare syrups in small quantities. Large quantities require incorporation of a preservative like methyl paraben, benzoic acid, or sodium benzoate.

Nowadays other sweetening agents such as saccharin sodium and cyclamates can be used in place of sucrose. However, it is necessary to include a thickening agent like sodium carboxy methyl cellulose to raise the viscosity in such cases.

3. Elixirs

Elixirs are clear, liquid oral preparations of potent or nauseous drugs such as antibiotics, antihistamines and sedatives, etc. They are pleasantly flavoured hydroalcoholic liquids. Clarity of elixirs can be achieved by selecting a suitable vehicle. Following are the main ingredients of elixirs :

(i) Vehicle

Suitable amount of alcohol, glycerin are added to prevent precipitation of various vegetable extracts, as phenobarbitone is insoluble in water but a clear product can be made by dissolving it in alcohol and then diluting with glycerol and water. The concentration of alcohol is always kept minimum to avoid its physiological activity. Paediatric elixirs do not contain alcohol. Flavoured syrups are generally added to it. The bitter and nauseous taste can be marked by flavouring and sweetening agent.

(ii) *Stabilizers*

Micro-organism growth cannot take place if elixirs contain more than 20% of alcohol, propylene glycol, or glycerol. Commonly used additional preservative is chloroform which is used in the form of double strength water, the spirit or the pure substance. Neomycin elixir is generally adjusted to pH 4 to 5 with citric acid to minimise the darkening on storage.

(iii) *Colouring agent*

Elixirs can be medicated or non-medicated. To provide colour to elixirs various colouring agents are used, e.g., amaranth, compound tartrazine, greens and tartrazine.

(iv) *Flavouring agent*

Flavouring agents are added to mask the nauseous taste and odour of certain drugs, e.g., compound orange spirit, black currant syrup, raspberry juice, lemon spirit.

(v) *Sweetening agent*

Bitter taste of drugs can be masked by making the preparation sweet with flavoured syrup. In addition to this, glycerin, sorbitol, and saccharin may be used. Saccharin helps in concealing the bitter taste of certain antibiotics.

LIQUIDS FOR EXTERNAL ADMINISTRATION OR USED ON MUCOUS MEMBRANE

Gargles

Gargles are aqueous solutions meant for treatment of an infection of pharynx and nasopharynx. Usually they are supplied in concentrated forms and must be diluted with water prior to use. The product should be labelled with instructions so that it cannot be taken for internal administration. They help in relieving soreness in mild throat infections. They include several ingredients like phenol in small concentration which gives anaesthetic effect. Potassium chlorate is added to provide weak astringent effect and to stimulate saliva. Thymol glycerin is another example in which alcohol is added to dissolve thymol, menthol, cineole, methyl salicylate. The alcoholic solution is then mixed with talc. It is then added to a solution containing borax, sodium bicarbonate, sodium benzoate, sodium metabisulphite and glycerin. Glycerin gives sweet taste to the preparation. Sodium metabisulphite is added to protect sodium salicylate.

While using gargles, the solution is brought into intimate contact with mucous membrane of throat and then they are allowed to remain there for a moment after which they are thrown out of the mouth cavity.

Mouth Washes

A mouthwash is an aqueous solution meant for cleaning, refreshing and deodorant action. They are generally pleasantly flavoured, coloured solutions containing antibacterial agents. Use of medicated mouth washes should always be guided under the supervision of dentist because they contain astringents and other medicaments whose continuous use may be harmful. Compound sodium chloride mouth wash is very common which contains sodium chloride, sodium bicarbonate in peppermint and chloroform water.

Throat Paints

Throat paints are liquid preparations meant for mouth and throat infections. They contain high concentration of glycerin which helps to prolong the contact time of the drug by making the preparation viscous. Glycerin provides a sweet taste to the preparations. In general, the drugs used are antibiotics, sulfonamides, iodides, phenol and tannic acid. Commonly used throat paints are boroglycerin, phenol glycerin, tannic acid glycerin and Mandle's paint. They are generally applied using a soft brush. Throat paints provide analgesic effect in tonsillitis while the astringent action of tannic acid glycerin relieves sore throat.

Douches

A douche is a medicated solution which is used for rinsing a body cavity. The word 'douche' is often used for vaginal solutions. Similarly vaginal solutions are also known as irrigations. Douches are meant for various purposes :

1. Antiseptics, e.g., mercuric chloride (0.001%), chlorhexidine (0.02%), potassium permanganate (0.025%).
2. Cleansing agent, e.g., isotonic solution of sodium chloride.
3. Astringents, e.g., alum (1%).

They are used to irrigate eyes, ear or nasal cavities to remove foreign particles.

Douches are generally dispensed in the form of a powder with specific directions for dissolution. 'Douche can' is used for this purpose which is fitted with a rubber tube of 2 metre length along with a nozzle. It can hold generally a solution of 1 litre to 2 litres.

Ear Drops

Ear drops are the liquid preparations which are meant for instillation into ear cavity to treat ear infections, etc. Various antibiotics (chloramphenicol, etc.) are used to treat acute infections of ear. Generally propylene glycol and glycerol are used as vehicles. Ear drops are used for softening the wax (sodium bicarbonate or hydrogen peroxide) and for cleansing the ear cavity. Phenol is sometimes added in small amounts to provide antiseptic and anaesthetic effect. A secondary label must be attached with a direction "For external use only.". Ear drops are dispensed in coloured fluted bottles attached with a dropper.

Nasal Drops and Spray

Nasal drops

Nasal drops are aqueous solutions which are meant for instillation into nasal cavity for their antiseptic, local analgesic and vasoconstrictor action.

Nasal drops should be isotonic with 0.9% sodium chloride. The buffering capacity of nasal mucous is quite low and strong alkaline solutions can cause considerable damage to cilia. Therefore it is advisable to use a phosphate buffer of pH 6.5 as a vehicle. The viscosity of these preparations can be achieved by adding 0.5% methylcellulose to it.

Nasal preparation must not interfere with the cleansing action of epithelial cilia of nasal mucosa.

In the past oily vehicles such as liquid paraffin and vegetable oils were used as vehicles for nasal drops but repeated use showed that it interferes with ciliary activity and produces lipoidal pneumonia. Nowadays they are dispensed in aqueous vehicles only. They are dispensed in coloured fluted bottles fitted with dropper and labelled with directions "Not to be taken." or "For use only in nose.".

Nasal sprays

Nasal sprays are used to reduce nasal congestion and to treat infections. The main purpose is to retain the droplets in the nasal tract, so for this purpose they are applied as a coarse spray into the nostrils. They are usually packed in flexible plastic containers with an orifice through which the liquid passes as a spray into nostril when the container is pressed. Some of the U.S.P. official nasal sprays are naphazoline hydrochloride, phenylephrine hydrochloride. Spray should be isotonic and buffered at pH 6.2. They may contain antibiotics, antihistamines, etc.

Liniment

Liniments are liquid or semi-liquid preparations meant for skin and are applied by rubbing to the affected area. Alcoholic liniments are generally used for their rubifacient, counterirritant, and mild astringent effects. Oily liniment (liniment with oil as a base) cannot penetrate the skin readily therefore they are slow in their action but are very useful while massaging. Liniments are always applied with friction on unbroken skin. They are usually meant for analgesic, rubifacient, soothing or stimulating properties. Example : camphor liniment is a solution of camphor in arachis oil, soap liniment is a solution of camphor in an alcoholic solution of soap which is formed in situ. The label must carry these instructions : "Not to be applied to wounds or broken skin." and "For external use only.". They should be stored in a cool place because volatile substances are present.

Lotion

Lotions are usually liquid suspensions or dispersions meant for external application and are applied gently on the affected area. They are usually antipruritic, astringent, analgesic, anaesthetic and emollient in action. They are applied to skin with the help of some cotton wool or gauze soaked in solution. The main ingredients are zinc sulphate, lead sub-acetate, etc., which are soluble in water. For salicylic acid, alcohol is added to dissolve it. Alcohol is sometimes added in aqueous lotion to produce cooling effect while glycerin keeps the skin moist for sufficiently long time and hastens the drying of preparation. Preservatives are added to lotions to prevent the growth of bacteria and moulds. All lotions are labelled "For external use only.". Lotions are dispensed in coloured fluted bottles to distinguish from preparations which are used for internal purposes. After some time, lotions have a tendency to separate out solids therefore they must be labelled with additional direction "Shake the bottle before use.".

6

Biphasic Liquid Dosage Form

Suspensions

Suspensions are the biphasic liquid dosage form of the medicament meant for oral administration, external application and for parenteral use. They generally consist of finely divided solid particles ranging from 0.5 to 5.0 μ suspended in a liquid or semi-solid vehicle.

The particle size of the disperse phase is an important consideration in the formulation process. The suspensions meant for topical application should have small particle size to avoid a gritty feel and to provide greater coverage of the area of application. If the solid substance is meant for skin penetration, its small size gives a faster rate of dissolution and therefore helps penetration. Injectable suspension should have a particle size that can pass through the needle. In suspensions meant for introduction into the ophthalmic cavity the particle size should not go beyond 10 μ. Suspension is an ideal dosage form for patients who cannot swallow tablets or capsules.

Qualities of Good Suspension

Suspension should have the following properties :

1. It should be chemically stable.
2. The sediment produced on standing should be easily redispersed.
3. The viscosity should be such that the preparation can be easily poured.
4. Suspensions meant for internal use must be palatable and suspensions for external use must be free from gritty particles.

(i) Suspensions containing diffusible solids

Solids which are insoluble in water but readily mix with water and remain suspended throughout the liquid for sufficiently long time after shaking are known as diffusible solids.

Examples : $CaCO_3$, light $MgCO_3$, magnesium trisilicate, rhubarb powder and light kaolin.

Method of preparation

1. Finely powder all the ingredients in mortar.
2. Mix it with enough vehicle to form a smooth cream.
3. Add more of the vehicle to make it pourable.
4. Examine the contents for foreign particles and if present pass through a piece of muslin.
5. Add any liquid ingredient, rinse the measures and mix well after each addition.
6. Add more of the vehicle to produce the required volume.
7. Transfer the finished product into bottle, cork, clean it and attach the label with direction "Shake the bottle before use.".

Example :

(i) *Rx*

   Magnesium sulphate
   Light magnesium carbonate
   Peppermint water

(ii) *Rx*

   Bismuth carbonate
   Chloroform water

(iii) *Rx*

   Calcium carbonate
   Magnesium carbonate
   Peppermint water

(ii) Suspension containing indiffusible solids

A solid is regarded as indiffusible when it will not remain uniformly distributed in the vehicle for sufficiently long time. To suspend the drug certain thickening agents are added.

Table 6.1. Examples of indiffusible solids

Used internally	Used externally
Aspirin	Calamine
Chalk	Hydrocortisone
Phenobarbitone	Sulphur
Sulphadimidine	Precipitated sulphur
Succinylsulphathiazole	Zinc oxide

A. Thickening Agents

Thickening agents are hydrophillic colloids which form colloidal dispersions with water and increase the viscosity of continuous phase so that the particles remain suspended for a sufficiently long time and it becomes easy to measure an accurate dosage.

Classification of Thickening Agents

I. Polysaccharides

(a) *Natural agents*

(i) **Gum acacia.** Acacia is a good protective colloid and suspending agent. It gives less satisfactory results unless combined with other thickeners like compound tragacanth powder (CPT). CPT is always used when the vehicle is other than chloroform water or water. It is generally used in the amount of 10 grains/oz of the mixture. It contains an oxidase enzyme that causes deterioration of easily oxidisable medicament. Therefore, antimicrobial substances like benzoic acid or parahydroxybenzoic acid are added.

(ii) **Tragacanth.** It is a much better thickening agent than acacia. It is used as powder (CPT) or as mucilage to suspend heavy indiffusible substances. It produces less sticky mucilage than acacia. Tragacanth mucilage is used when the vehicle is water or chloroform and only 1/4th of the volume of mixture is used.

(iii) **Starch.** It is used with other suspending agents because of the high viscosity of its mucilage. It is an ingredient of compound tragacanth powder (2%).

(iv) **Sodium alginate.** It forms a viscous solution with water where about 1 per cent gives a product with approximately the same suspending powder as tragacanth mucilage. The viscosity of alginate mucilage shows a fall after 24 hours. Therefore, they should be allowed to stand overnight before using them. It is otherwise incompatible with heavy metals and calcium salts.

(b) *Semi-synthetic*

Cellulose derivatives

Methylcellulose is used in both internal and external preparations where the concentration depends on the viscosity of the polymer but is usually between 0.5 and 2%. Sodium carboxymethyl cellulose is more sensitive to pH than methylcellulose. It is used in concentration from 0.25 to 1% as suspending agent in parenteral, oral and external products. Microcrystalline cellulose is prepared from wood cellulose by acid hydrolysis. It is not soluble in water. It swells and partly dissolves in dilute alkali.

II. Inorganic agents

(a) *Clays*

Several natural clays like bentonite and aluminium magnesium silicate are used as thickening agents.

Bentonite, a dispersion containing 2% bentonite, is suitable for suspending indiffusible solids. It should be sterilised before use because it may contain *Clostridium tetani*. Aluminium and magnesium silicate (common name vecgum) is used in concentration of 0.5 to 2%.

(b) *Aluminium hydroxide*

It is sometimes used as a suspending agent for $BaSO_4$, calamine, sulphur, etc.

III. Synthetic agents

Carbomer (carboxy vinyl polymer). It is used as a thickening agent for external and internal preparation in very low concentration (0.5-0.4%).

Colloidal silicon dioxide. It acts as a thickening agent because when suspended in a liquid, the particles associate due to hydrogen bonding. About 12% gives a soft gel with water but 1.5 to 4% is enough to stabilise suspension.

B. Wetting Agents

Wetting agents are added to prepare suspensions of desired quality by reducing interfacial tension between the solid particles and liquid medium. Wetting agent gets absorbed at the solid/liquid interface in such a way that the affinity of the particles for the surrounding medium is increased and the interparticular forces are decreased. Excessive use of wetting agent may cause foaming or may give bad taste or odour to the preparation.

Examples :

   (i)   Alcohol in tragacanth mucilage.

  (ii)   Glycerin and glycols in sodium alginate dispersion.

 (iii)   Polysorbates in oral and parenteral suspensions.

Method of preparation (using compound tragacanth powder CPT)

   1.   Finely powder all the ingredients. Mix them with CPT thoroughly. To this add 3/4th of vehicle slowly, so as to form a smooth cream.

2. Examine the contents for foreign particles, if present pass the contents through muslin cloth and rinse the mortar with little bit of vehicle.
3. Add any liquid ingredient, i.e., mix and finally add more of vehicle to produce the final volume.
4. Transfer the suspension into bottle with a direction on label "Shake well before use.".

When we use tragacanth mucilage as suspending agent, mix all the indiffusible solids, diffusible solids and soluble solids with tragacanth mucilage (1/4th of the mixture) and 1/2 of the vehicle to form a smooth cream. The product will then measure 3/4th of the vehicle.

(iii) Suspensions of precipitate forming liquids

In case of liquid preparations containing resinous substances resin therein gets precipitated and may adhere to the side of the bottle which will not diffuse upon shaking. Hence compound tragacanth powder or tragacanth mucilage is used.

Examples : compound benzoin tincture, benzoin tincture, myrrh tincture, tincture tolu.

Method of preparation (by using compound tragacanth powder)

1. Finely powder the indiffusible solid, and diffusible solid in the mortar and mix intimately with CPT.
2. Triturate the mixture with the vehicle to form a smooth cream and dilute gradually to about 50 per cent of the final volume.
3. Measure precipitate forming liquid in a measure and add it to the centre of suspension.
4. If the suspension contains an electrolyte,
   (i) it should be well diluted to about half of the remaining vehicle;
   (ii) it should be added slowly with constant stirring.
5. Observe the contents for foreign particles. If present, filter it.
   Steps 5, 6 and 7 are same as in the case of indiffusible mixture.

Method using tragacanth mucilage

(TM is used when the vehicle is water or chloroform water.)

1. Mix the mucilage with an equal volume of vehicle.
2. Measure precipitate forming liquid in a dry measure and pour slowly into the centre of the mucilage with rapid stirring. Dissolve any solid in about 1/4th of the vehicle and mix them.

(iv) Suspensions prepared by chemical reaction

If dilute solution of reactants are mixed, a fine diffusible precipitate is obtained by chemical reaction. Reacting substances are dissolved separately in approximately half volume of the vehicle and the two parts are mixed, e.g.,

> Zinc sulphide lotion B.P.C.
>
> Sulphurated potash
>
> Zinc sulphate
>
> Concentrated camphor water
>
> Water

Procedure

(i) Dissolve sulphurated potash and $ZnSO_4$ separately in small quantity of vehicle.

(ii) Add sulphurated potash slowly to the zinc sulphate solution with rapid stirring.

(iii) Transfer to a tared container.

(iv) Add camphor water with vigorous shaking to redissolve precipitated camphor.

(v) Mix it well and make up the volume.

Flocculated and Non-flocculated Suspensions

The suspensions are said to be flocculated when the individual particles are in contact with each other and form a network-like structure, and are said to be deflocculated, if every individual particle exists as a separate entity. Following are the differences between flocculated and non-flocculated suspensions :

S. No.	Flocculated suspensions	Non-flocculated suspensions
1.	Particles form a loose aggregate.	Particles exist as separate entities.
2.	Since it is an aggregate of particles so rate of sedimentation is quicker.	Particles settle down and rate of sedimentation is slow.
3.	Sediment is loosely packed.	Sediment is closely packed and hard cake is formed.
4.	Sediment is easy to redisperse.	Sediment is difficult to redisperse.
5.	Supernatant liquid is clear.	Supernatant liquid is not clear.
6.	Floccules stick to the sides of the bottle.	They do not stick to the sides of the bottle.

Emulsion

An emulsion is a biphasic liquid dosage form of two immiscible liquids, one of which is distributed in the form of fine globules in the other liquid. They are made miscible by the addition of a third substance known as emulsifying agent. The liquid that is broken up into globules is called the dispersed phase or internal phase and the liquid in which the globules are dispersed is known as continuous or external phase.

Advantages

(i) Medicines having objectionable odour and taste (castor oil) can be made more palatable for oral administration when formulated in an emulsion.

(ii) Cream, lotion and foam aerosols are formulated in emulsion.

(iii) Absorption, penetration, therapeutic effect and spreadability of the constituent can be increased.

(iv) Emulsion provides protection against drugs susceptible to oxidation or hydrolysis.

(v) I.V. emulsion of contrast media have been developed to assist the doctor in understanding x-ray examination of body organs while exposing the patient to the minimum of radiation.

Types of Emulsions

Emulsions are of two types :

(i) Oil in water type (o/w)

(ii) Water in oil type (w/o)

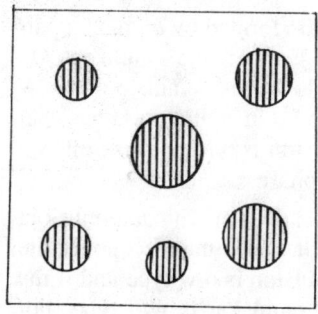
O/w emulsion

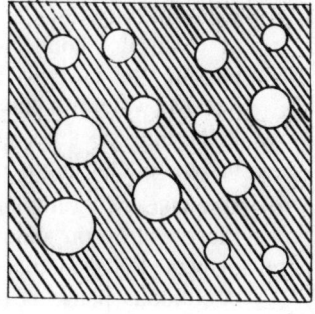
W/o emulsion

Fig. 6.1.

Oil in water (o/w)	Water in oil (w/o)
1. Oil is in the dispersed phase and water in the continuous phase.	Water is in the dispersed phase and oil in the continuous phase.
2. O/w emulsions can be easily removed and evaporation of water causes cooling effect.	W/o emulsions prevent dehydration from the skin and provide emollient effect.
3. Water soluble medicaments are more quickly released from o/w emulsions.	Oil soluble medicaments are released more quickly from w/o emulsions.
4. O/w emulsions are preferred for internal use because the unpleasant taste can be masked and water is in the external phase.	W/o emulsions are mainly used externally as lotions or creams.
5. Emulsifying agents like gum, acacia, tragacanth, methyl cellulose, and soaps formed from monovalent bases like Na^+, K^+, and NH_4^+ are used.	Emulsifying agents like wool fat, resins, bees wax and soaps formed from divalent bases like Ca^{++}, Mg^{++} and Zn^{++} are used for the preparation of water in oil emulsion.

Identification of Emulsion System

As both o/w and w/o emulsions are similar in appearance therefore to determine the type of emulsion, following tests are performed :

(i) **Dilution test.** Take 5-10 drops of emulsion in a test tube and dilute with 2-3 drops of water. If emulsion gets mixed with water then it is of o/w type but if water separates then the emulsion is of w/o type. Similarly on dilution with oil, the oil distributes itself uniformly in w/o emulsion and separates out in o/w emulsion.

(ii) **Conductivity test.** This test can be performed by dipping a pair of electrodes connected through a lamp in the emulsion. On passing the current, if the bulb glows, the emulsion is o/w because water is a good conductor and is in continuous phase but if the bulb does not glow, the emulsion is w/o because oil is a bad conductor and is in continuous phase.

(iii) **Dye test.** Mix oil-soluble dye like scarlet red with an emulsion. Place a drop on slide and observe it under microscope. If the dispersed phase is red in colour, emulsion is o/w type and if the continuous phase is red in colour, emulsion is w/o type. For confirmation this test can be repeated with water-soluble dye amaranth. With this dispersed phase will appear to be red in w/o emulsion and continuous phase will appear to be red in o/w emulsion.

Formulation of Emulsion

Formulation of emulsion requires following to be decided critically :

(i) Oily phase

(ii) Aqueous phase

(iii) Emulsifying agent or emulgent

(i) **Oily phase** should be

Non-toxic

Non-irritant

Stable

Compatible

Of optimum consistency

(ii) **Aqueous phase** should be

Free from dissolved solids

Free from ions

Free from foreign particles

(iii) **Emulsifying agents — emulgents or emulsifiers**

Emulsifying agents reduce the interfacial tension between oil and water and thus help in the dispersion of one liquid in the other.

Selection

1. It should be physically and chemically stable.
2. It should be non-toxic.
3. It should be compatible with the preparation.
4. It should reduce the interfacial tension between the two phases.
5. It should be capable of maintaining the required viscosity of the emulsion.

Griffin has provided a logical means of selecting an emulgent, called 'Hydrophillic Lipophillic Balance'. HLB scale is divided into 18 units. More polar and hydrophillic compounds have a higher HLB value. If the surfactant has a low HLB value (3.5-6.0) it will produce w/o emulsion but if the surfactant has high HLB value (8-18) it will produce o/w emulsions. To achieve stable emulsion it is therefore advisable to use mixture of two surfactants. Desirable HLB of emulsifying agents for o/w emulsion ranges between 8-18 and that for w/o emulsions from 3-6.

Table 6.2. Classification of emulsifying agents

Name	Concentration	Properties
1. Natural emulsifying agent (from veg. sources)		
Gum acacia	8-15%	It gives stable and emulsions of palatable taste over pH range (2-10). Viscosity is low, may cause creaming which can be prevented by adding agar, tragacanth.
Tragacanth	1-2%	Rarely used, because it gives very coarse and thick emulsions. Appearance and stability can be improved by passing through a homogenizer.
Agar	2%	Below 45°C it will form a gel which is not suitable for emulsion. The mucilage is added in the primary emulsion in sufficient quantity to make 30 to 50 per cent of the final volume.
Irish moss (chondrus)	3%	solution with an equal volume of oil Like agar, it is not a primary emulsifier but is used as thickening agent. It is used along with acacia for the emulsification of cod-liver oil.
Pectin	1%	It acts as an emulsion stabiliser in acacia emulsions. Incompatible with alkalies, strong alcohol, tannic and salicylic acid.
Starch	2-5%	Rarely used because it forms very coarse emulsions.
2. Natural emulsifying agent (from animal sources)		
Gelatin	1%	Pharmagol A — acidic pH Pharmagol B — alkaline pH Emulsions are of agreeable taste but prone to bacterial growth so preservative is added.
Egg yolk	12-15%	Mainly used for extemporaneous preparations because emulsions get spoiled during transportation. It should be stored in a refrigerator.
Wool fat (anhydrous lanolin)	20%	Meant for external use emulsions and can absorb 50% of water. It may lead to allergic manifestation.

Contd.

Name	Concentration	Properties

3. Semi-synthetic polysaccharides

Name	Concentration	Properties
Methyl cellulose	2%	It is used widely as suspending, thickening and emulsifying agent, stable over wide range of pH. Mainly used for emulsification of mineral and vegetable oil but get precipitated in the presence of large amount of electrolytes.
Sodium carboxy methyl cellulose	0.5-1%	True emulsifier, emulsion stabilizer. It is soluble in cold water, hot water. Compatible with up to 40% of alcohol content.

4. Synthetic emulsifying agent

Name	Concentration	Properties
Surface active agents	(i) Anionic	Various alkali soaps, metallic soaps, sulphated alcohols are used as E.A. soap. Emulsions are not stable at pH values less than 10.
	(ii) Cationic	Examples : benzalkonium chloride, cetrimide. Mainly used for external use preparations.
	(iii) Non-ionic	Examples : glyceryl monostearate, sorbitan monopalminate. Widely used because remain stable over wide range of pH changes.

5. Inorganic emulsifying agent

Name	Concentration	Properties
Milk of magnesia	10-20%	Gives coarse emulsion. Mainly used for mineral oil emulsions.
Magnesium oxide	5-10%	Gives coarse emulsion. Mainly used for mineral oil emulsions.
Magnesium aluminium silicate	1%	Compatible with alcohol over a wide pH range.
Bentonite	5%	Used to prepare o/w or w/o emulsions. For the preparation of o/w emulsion oil is added to the suspension of bentonite whereas in w/o emulsions the oil is placed in the container and bentonite suspensions is added to the oil.

6. Alcohols

Name	Concentration	Properties
Cholesterol	(i) Cetyl alcohol Stearyl alcohol	Rarely used.

Contd.

Name	Concentration	Properties
(ii) Carbo-waxes	Mol. wt. — 200-700 (viscous liquids) Mol. wt. — 1000 and above (solids). A product of desired consistency can be obtained.

Preparation of Emulsions

Emulsions can be prepared by the following methods :

    (i) Dry gum method
   (ii) Wet gum method
  (iii) Bottle method
  (iv) Other methods

Primary Emulsion

Measure the quantity of oil/water triturated with calculated quantity of gum acacia to form a uniform mixture. Then add required quantity of water/oil accordingly with rapid trituration until a clicking sound is produced and the product becomes white due to the total internal reflection of light. At this stage, the emulsion is known as primary emulsion.

Table 6.3. Ratio of oil, water and gum acacia required for fixed, volatile and mineral oils (ratio for primary emulsion)

Type of oil	Examples	Oil	Water	Gum
Fixed	Almond oil, arachis oil, castor oil, cod-liver oil	4	2	1
Volatile	Turpentine oil, cinnamon oil, peppermint oil	2	2	1
Mineral	Liquid paraffin	3	2	1

(i) Dry gum method (4 : 2 : 1 method)

1. Measure oil with a dry measuring cylinder and transfer it into a dry mortar.
2. Add calculated quantity of gum acacia to it and triturate rapidly so as to form a uniform mixture.
3. Add required quantity of water to form a primary emulsion and triturate vigorously till a clicking sound is produced.
4. Add more of water to produce the final volume. If any soluble ingredient is to be added it must be incorporated after making the primary emulsion.

(ii) Wet gum method

It gives less good results than the dry gum method.

Procedure

1. Calculated quantity of gum acacia is triturated with measured quantity of water to form a mucilage.
2. To this add oil in small portions with rapid trituration until the product becomes white and clicking sound is produced.
3. When primary emulsion is formed, add more of the vehicle to produce the final volume.

(iii) Bottle method

This method is generally used for volatile oil. As volatile oils are less viscous, therefore they require greater amount of gum acacia for their emulsification (4 : 4 : 2).

Procedure

1. Put the oil in a bottle, add gum acacia to it.
2. Bottle is shaken vigorously for some time.
3. Add calculated amount of water all at once.
4. Mixture is shaken vigorously to form a primary emulsion.
5. Add more of water with constant agitation to produce the required volume.

(vi) Other methods

Various homogenisers and blenders can be used for preparing emulsions.

(i) *Kenwood mixer*

It is used for small batches of emulsions. The mixing action is planetary which reaches all the liquid in the mixing vessel and not just the centre portion (ordinary mixing).

(ii) *Silverson mixer-emulsifier*

It consists of a stainless steel working head containing rotor blades for emulsification. The head is suspended so that it can be immersed in the liquids to be emulsified. High speed rotation is given and material is expelled through the sieve.

(iii) *Hand homogeniser*

This homogeniser is hand operated and the coarse emulsion is passed through a fine orifice. The emulsion is placed in the hopper of the homogeniser. The up and down movement of the handle causes coarse emulsion to draw in through homogenising valve and the emulsion passes through fine orifice and oil globules. The emulsion finally gets broken into fine globules of uniform size.

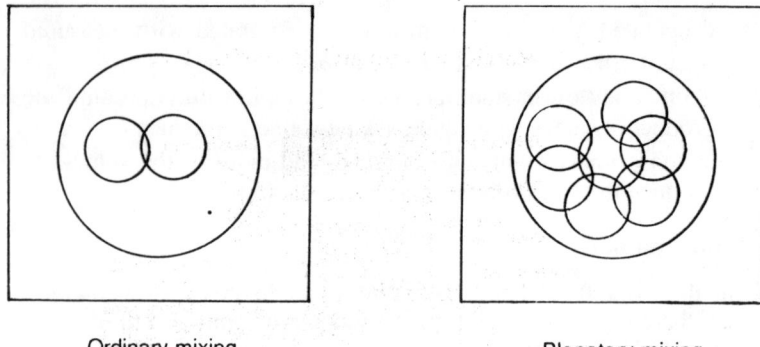

Ordinary mixing   Planetary mixing

Fig. 6.2.

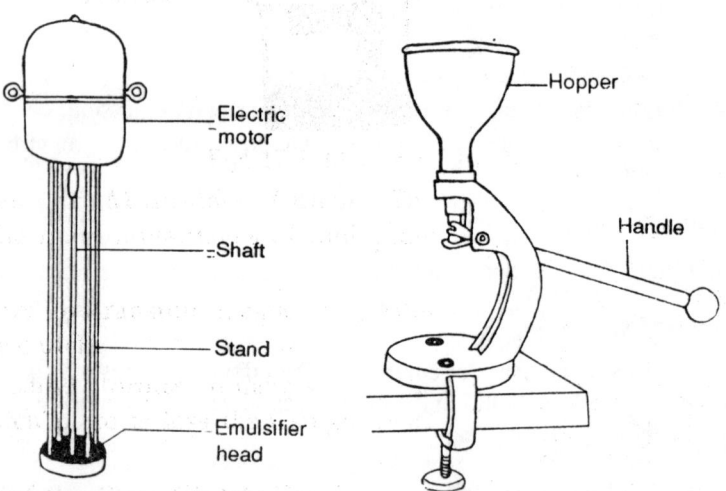

Fig. 6.3. Silverson mixer homogeniser.   **Fig. 6.4.** Hand homogeniser.

Instabilities in Emulsions

There are three major factors which are responsible for instabilities in emulsions :

1. Cracking
2. Creaming
3. Phase inversion

1. Cracking

Cracking refers to the separation of two layers of disperse and continuous phases due to the coalescence of disperse phase globules which are difficult to redisperse by shaking.

Cracking may be due to the following reasons :

(i) *Addition of an emulgent of opposite type :* Soaps of monovalent metals produce o/w emulsions while soaps of divalent metals produce w/o emulsions. But the addition of a monovalent soap to a divalent soap emulsion or a divalent soap to a monovalent soap emulsion leads to cracking.

(ii) *Decomposition or precipitation of emulsifying agent :*

   (a) Addition of alcohol to the liniment of turpentine dissolves the soft soap which is the emulsifying agent.

   (b) The addition of sodium chloride to sodium soap emulsion precipitates the emulsifying agent and causes cracking.

   (c) Changes in temperature : When emulsions are stored for sufficiently long time, an increase in temperature may reduce viscosity of emulsion and encourage creaming. Freezing may lead to the water in the emulsion being converted into ice. Subsequent melting of the ice and shaking may not reform the emulsion.

   (d) Addition of a common solvent : Addition of a liquid which can dissolve the disperse phase, continuous phase and the emulsifying agent will form a clear monophasic system thus destroying the emulsion, e.g., alcohol in turpentine oil liniment may form a clear solution because alcohol is miscible with turpentine oil, water, and soft soap.

   (e) Microbial action : If the emulsions are not stored properly they may develop mould growth which may destroy the emulsifying agent and cause cracking.

2. Creaming

Creaming may be defined as the formation of concentrated layer of disperse globules at the surface of emulsion (e.g., milk o/w) whereas in sedimentation dispersed globules move downwards and form a thick layer at the bottom. Creaming is undesirable but it is a temporary phase which can be redistributed by mild shaking. According to Stoke's law following are the ways to minimise creaming :

$$V = \frac{2r^2 (d_1 - d_2) g}{9n}$$

where V = rate of creaming

r = radius of globules

d_1 = density of dispersed phase

d_2 = density of continuous phase

g = gravitational constant

n = viscosity of the dispersion medium.

Creaming of emulsions can be reduced by adopting following methods :

1. *Size reduction of globule*

Rate of creaming is directly related to size of globules. Larger the size, more will be the creaming and smaller the size lesser will be the creaming. Small globules will rise less quickly than large globules. Hence, effective homogenisation will reduce the size of globules.

2. *Increasing the viscosity of continuous phase*

As rate of creaming is inversely proportional to the viscosity of continuous phase, viscosity can be increased by adding tragacanth and sodium alginate with affecting densities of continuous phase.

3. *Storage condition*

As high temperature reduces viscosity which may lead to creaming therefore emulsions should be stored in a cool place. Freezing of aqueous phase should be avoided which may lead to cracking.

3. **Phase inversion (inversion of phase o/w → w/o)**

Phase inversion means the change of one type of emulsion into the other type, i.e., o/w type emulsion changes into w/o type and vice versa. It may be due to following reasons :

  (i) By addition of an electrolyte

  (ii) By changing phase-volume ratio

  (iii) By changing emulsifying agent

  (iv) By temperate change.

Phase volume ratio is an important factor. If the concentration of disperse phase is less than 30% it may lead to creaming and if it is more than 60% particularly more than 75% it may cause phase inversion. Therefore the most stable range of disperse phase concentration is 30 to 60 per cent.

Preservation of Emulsions

1. Preservation against micro-organisms

Emulsions get contaminated by micro-organisms which may cause unpleasant odour, discoloration and due to breakdown of the emulsifying agent, changes occur in consistency also. Therefore antimicrobial agents are added.

Properties of antimicrobial substances

1. It should be effective against wide range of microorganisms.
2. It should be non-toxic.
3. It should be odourless and tasteless.
4. It should preserve the preparation and remain stable for a long time.
5. It should be compatible with all the ingredients.

Table 6.4.

Name of the preservative	Concentration	Properties
1. Benzoic acid	0.1-0.2% pH (< 5.0)	Ant.fungal, antibacterial.
2. Methyl paraben and propyl paraben	0.1-0.2%	Stable, inert, non-toxic, active against moulds, yeast and bacteria.
3. Sorbic acid	0.1-0.2%	Effective at pH 6.5. Used for acacia and tragacanth mucilage.
4. Chloroform	0.25%	It is used with benzoic acid in liquid paraffin emulsion.
5. Chlorocresol	0.1%	Powerful bactericide for aqueous creams. Activity gets reduced in alkaline solution.
6. Cetrimide	0.002-0.01%	Bactericide for emulsified products of external use.
7. Phenyl mercuric	0.004-0.01%	To preserve emulsified nitrate preparations containing non-ionic emulgents.

2. Preservation from atmospheric oxygen

Antioxidants are added to prevent oxidative degradation of fat and oil of animal and vegetable origin by competitive inhibition mechanism. Anti-oxidant used for this purpose should have following properties :

1. It should be physically and chemically stable.
2. It should be effective against wide range of pH.
3. It should be non-toxic and non-irritant.
4. It should be thermostable.
5. It should be compatible with other ingredients of formulation.

Table 6.5. Examples of anti-oxidants and their properties

Name of the anti-oxidant	Properties
1. Tocopherol	Natural antioxidant, used for vit. A emulsions.
2. BHT (butylated hydroxy toluene)	For preservation of fats, fixed BHA (butylated hydroxy anisole) and volatile oil.
3. Pyragallol	For fixed oils and fats.
4. Gallic acid	To stabilise paraldehyde.
5. Propyl gallate	0.01% for fats, fixed oils; 0.05% for paraldehyde. Less toxic.
6. Ascorbic acid	For emulsified fats and oils.

7
Ointments

Definition

Ointments are semi-solid preparations meant for external application to the skin or mucous membrane. They are used for emollient, protective or other surface effects or they may contain medicaments which are to be absorbed systemically.

Accordingly they are classified as :

(i) Epidermatic — meant for action on epidermis;

(ii) Endodermatic — meant for action on deeper layers of cutaneous tissues;

(iii) Diadermatic — meant to penetrate deep and release medicaments to body fluids.

They can also be classified according to their use, e.g., protectives, counter-irritants, astringents, antiseptic ointments, etc.

Classification of Dermatological Vehicles

There are four main types of dermatological vehicles :

1. Oleaginous bases
2. Absorption bases
3. Water miscible bases
4. Water soluble bases

Table 7.1.

S. No.	Name of the base	Properties
1.	**Oleaginous bases or hydrocarbon bases**	Greasy and consist of water insoluble hydrophobic oils and fats, retain body heat. They are not absorbed by skin. Inert, cheap and readily available. They are sticky in nature.

Contd.

S. No.	Name of the base	Properties
(a)	Petrolatum (soft paraffin)	It is a purified mixture of semi-solid hydro-carbons obtained from petroleum. M.P. 38°C to 56°C. Translucent. Two varieties : one is yellow and the other, a bleached form, white. White soft paraffin is used when the medicament is white/colourless. Being inert, they are not absorbed, and therefore suitable for epidermal preparations. They have hydrophobic nature, so aqueous liquids cannot be mixed with it but sometimes wool fat and waxes are added to incorporate aqueous liquids in it.
(b)	Hard paraffin	This is a mixture of solid hydrocarbons obtained from petroleum. Colourless, odourless, tasteless, translucent, wax-like substance. It is used to stiffen the ointment base. Solidifies between 50°C and 57°C.
(c)	Liquid paraffin or liquid petrolatum or white mineral oil	This is a mixture of liquid hydrocarbons obtained from petroleum. Odourless, colourless, tasteless, oily liquid, insoluble in water and alcohol but soluble in ether and $CHCl_3$. Used with other paraffins to obtain desired consistency.
2.	**Absorption bases**	Hydrophillic nature. Water soluble. Can absorb large quantity of water. Compatible with large number of drugs. Heat stable. Good solvent properties. These bases have undesirable property of greasiness but they can be more easily removed from the skin as compared to the oily bases.
(a)	Wool fat or anhydrous lanolin	Purified anhydrous fat-like substance obtained from the wool of sheep. It can absorb 50% of its weight of water but it is too sticky to be used as a base. It is an important constituent of simple ointment base and eye ointment base.
(b)	Hydrous wool fat or lanolin	Purified fat-like substance obtained from wool of sheep. Insoluble in water but soluble in ether and $CHCl_3$. It is prepared from wool fat (70%) and water (30%). It is used alone as emollient and ingredient of several other ointments.

Contd.

S. No.	Name of the base	Properties
	(c) Wool alcohol	It is obtained from wool fat by treating it with alkali and separating the fraction containing cholesterol and other alcohols. It contains not less than 30% of cholesterol. It is used to improve stability of o/w emulsions. It acts as an emulsifying agent. :
	(d) Bees wax	Purified wax obtained from honeycomb of bees. Two varieties : one is yellow and the other, a bleached form, is white. It is used as a stiffening agent in pastes, ointments.
3.	**Water miscible bases**	Can be easily washed. No interference with skin function. Good contact with skin due to surfactant contents. Miscible with exudates from lesions. Cosmetic acceptability. Used for preparing o/w creams and for other ointments. There are three official anhydrous water miscible bases : the emulsifying ointment, i.e., emulsifying ointment B.P. — anionic; cetrimide emulsifying ointment B.P. — cationic; cetomacrogol emulsifying ointment — non-ionic. They contain paraffins, an o/w emulgent and have the general formula : White soft paraffin 50% Liquid paraffin 20% Appropriate anionic, cationic or non-ionic 30% emulsifying wax.
4.	**Water soluble bases or greaseless base**	They contain water soluble ingredients. Can be easily washed from the skin. Good absorption by skin. Good solvent properties.. Compatible with large number of drugs. Limited uptake of water. They may reduce activity of certain antibacterial agents. Water soluble bases are popularly known as carbowaxes (polyethylene glycol polymers or macrogols). They are non-volatile and non-toxic and non-irritating to the skin. Their molecular weight varies from 200-8000. Macrogols 200, 300, 400 — viscous liquids Macrogols 1500 — semi-solid Macrogols 1500, 3000, 4000, 6000 — waxy solids.

Selection of Dermatological Vehicles

Following are the characteristics of an ideal ointment base :

1. It should be stable and non-irritating.
2. It should be easily removable from the skin.
3. It should release the medicament easily.
4. It should be miscible with the skin secretions and with medicaments.
5. It should be inert, smooth and non-sensitizing.

Since there is no ointment base which satisfies all the above requirements, different ointment bases to suit different purposes are used. The factors which may help in the selection of an ideal ointment base are discussed below :

1. Dermatological factors
2. Pharmaceutical factors

1. Dermatological factors

(a) *Absorption and penetration*

The skin has three main layers : the epidermis, dermis and hypodermis. Penetration means passage through the skin whereas absorption means the actual entry into the blood. It is the ointment base that penetrates deep into the tissues of the skin along with the medicament and which in turn allows the systemic absorption of the medicament into the blood stream.

It is believed that animal fats (lard and wool fat) and oil penetrate readily through the skin, while mineral oils (paraffin) do not. Substances which are soluble both in oil and water are most readily absorbed. O/w emulsion bases release the medicament more readily than greasy bases or w/o emulsion bases. Paraffin bases have the least capability of releasing the medicament.

(b) *Effects on skin function*

Greasy bases may interfere with the skin functions and also irritate the skin, while o/w emulsion bases provide a cooling effect due to presence of water in their continuous phase.

(c) *Miscibility with skin secretions and serum*

Emulsion bases are more readily miscible with the skin aqueous or fatty secretions than the greasy bases. This miscibility results in a more rapid and complete release of medicament to the skin. Thus less medicament is necessary when such bases are used. O/w emulsions mix more readily with the serum from broken surfaces. They have also been found useful in pathological conditions.

(d) *Compatibility with skin secretions*

As the pH of skin is 5.5, the selection of the ointment base should be such that it is compatible with the skin as well as the medicament. Generally neutral ointment bases are selected.

(e) *Freedom from irritant effect*

Most of the bases are non-irritant except greasy bases. Ionic substances are also found to be irritant and even paraffins in emulsified form when they penetrate through the skin, may be harmful. So all bases used should be of high standard of purity specially for eye ointments.

(f) *Emollient properties*

Under normal conditions continuous hydration occurs which keeps the skin sufficiently moist but if dehydration occurs it results in dryness and brittleness. This causes discomfort and therefore humectants like glycerin and other hygroscopic substances can be incorporated to keep the surface soft and moist. Ointments containing wool fat, hard paraffin and liquid paraffin also act as emollient by preventing rapid loss of moisture from the skin.

(g) *Ease of application and removal*

This is an important factor to be considered otherwise it may cause damage to the newly formed tissues of skin. Therefore, emulsion bases are more preferred.

2. Pharmaceutical factors

(a) *Stability*

Fats and oils obtained from animal and vegetable sources are liable to undergo oxidation unless they are suitably preserved.

Table 7.2.

Name of the substance	Preservative
Lard	Butylated hydroxy toluene
Liquid paraffins	Butylated hydroxy toluene, tocopherol
Wool alcohols	Butylated hydroxy anisole

Soft paraffin, simple ointment and paraffin ointment are inert and stable. O/w type creams present a good medium for the growth of micro-organisms. Hence preservative should be added.

(b) *Solvent properties*

Most of the medicaments are insoluble in ointment bases therefore they should be present in fine form of powder so that it can be dispersed uniformly throughout the base. However, this may not be satisfactory for all the cases, e.g., phenol in solid form is caustic but finely divided powder form may cause blisters. Hence in phenol ointment B.P. the base is a mixture of hard and soft paraffin, bees wax and lard (lard ensures solution of phenol) while as in case of camphorated mercury ointment B.P.C. appreciable amount of olive oil is added to maintain camphor in the solution form.

(c) *Emulsifying properties*

Hydrocarbon bases cause poor water absorption resulting in poor emulsifying properties. While animal fats can absorb water to a great extent, e.g., wool fat can take up about 50% of water and when mixed with soft paraffin or lard it can take up several times its own weight of aqueous or hydroalcoholic liquids. For this reason wool fat is used in eye ointments.

Emulsifying ointment, cetrimide emulsifying ointment and ceto-macrogol emulsifying ointment are capable of absorbing considerable amount of water forming o/w creams.

(d) *Consistency*

The ointment should be of suitable consistency, neither too hard nor too soft. It should be able to withstand the temperature changes. Thus in summer, they should not become too soft and in winter not too hard to be difficult to use.

The consistency and rheological properties are adjusted by adding suitable amount of high melting point substances like hard paraffin, bees wax, etc., in soft ointments. Low melting point substances like liquid paraffins are used in hard ointments respectively.

Preparation of ointments

Ointments can be prepared by following methods :

1. Trituration method
2. Fusion method
3. Chemical reaction method
4. Emulsification method

1. Trituration method

This method is used when the base is soft and the medicament is insoluble in the base or a liquid is present in a small quantity.

Method

(i) Finely powder the solid ingredient if not already done.

(ii) Weigh out the required amount of base, add a portion of it on an ointment slab with the help of a stainless steel spatula and triturate thoroughly with drug until a homogenous product is formed.

(iii) Add remaining quantities of the base until the medicament is homogeneously mixed with the base and incorporate any liquid ingredient if present. When large volumes of liquid are to be added, pestle and mortar should be used for mixing. If the latter method is used, the sides of pestle and mortar should be scrapped from time to time. Further, there is a possibility of improper mixing of particles due to incomplete contact by this method leading to non-homogeneous product, e.g., zinc oxide ointment, sulphur ointment B.P.

2. Fusion method

When an ointment base contains several ingredients of different melting points, it is necessary to melt them in decreasing order of their melting points. This will avoid the overheating of substances having low melting point. The medicament is added slowly to the melted mass until a homogenous product is formed. This ensures that localised cooling does not occur. Rapid cooling will take place by transferring this mass into another container, cooling it under tap water and using a cold spatula.

Stirrer should be avoided in order to avoid the formation of solid lumps. Rapid cooling may result in separation of waxy solids and in such instances a homogenous product can be obtained by melting over low heat. Due to the greasy nature of ointment bases they pick up dirt during storage. This can be removed by allowing the melt to sediment and decanting the supernatant solution or by passing it through muslin cloth, e.g., simple ointment I.P.

3. Ointments prepared by chemical reaction

Chemical reactions are involved in the preparation of several ointments, e.g., iodine ointment. Iodine may be present in two forms :

(i) free

(ii) combined.

(i) *Ointments containing free iodine*

Iodine is slightly soluble in most fats and oils, but is readily soluble in KI solution forming polyiodides (KII_2, KI_2I_2, KI_3I_3). These polyiodides are rapidly soluble in water, alcohol and glycerin. In using a liquid to ensure proper distribution of a medicament, it is important that the liquid should be non-volatile, otherwise the distributed medicament may crystallize when the solvent evaporates.

(ii) *Ointments containing combined iodine*

All fixed oils and fats can absorb iodine which combines with the double bonds of unsaturated components, e.g.,

$$CH_3 (CH_2)_7CH\!\!=\!\!(CH_2)_7 \cdot COOH + I_2 = CH_3 (CH_2)_7 \cdot CHI \cdot CHI \cdot (CH_2)_7 \cdot COOH$$
$$\text{Oleic acid} \qquad \text{Iodine} \qquad \text{Di-iodo stearic acid}$$

Non-staining iodine ointment B.P.C.

Formula :

> Iodine
>
> Arachis oil
>
> Yellow soft paraffin

This preparation is dark, greenish black in colour and when rubbed onto the skin is readily absorbed and leaves no stains. Hence it is non-staining ointment.

Method of preparation

1. Finely powder the iodine and add the required amount to the oil in a glass stoppered conical flask.
2. Heat on a water bath at a temperature not exceeding 60°C. Brown colour will turn into greenish black. The time required for this may vary from 2-6 hrs.
3. Warm the yellow soft paraffin, add the iodised oil and mix well.
4. Pour into a warm pot of light resistant glass and allow it to cool.

4. Emulsification method

In this the fatty component is melted and the aqueous phase containing water soluble ingredient is also raised to the same temperature. The two phases are triturated well and the mixture is allowed to cool to form a semi-solid mass. This procedure is for ointment emulsions in which the emulsifying agent is formed in situ by reaction between a fatty acid and a suitable base such as borax or triethanolamine (e.g., vanishing cream).

Instead of forming the emulsifying agent in situ, which is usually a soap (cationic, anionic, non-ionic), emulsifying agents may be added to make ointment emulsion. Aqueous cream is an example.

Stability of Ointments

A stable ointment is one which retains its consistency throughout its shelf life. The main stability problems are as follows :

1. Bleeding

When fluid component separates at the top of the ointment, the phenomenon is called bleeding.

2. Change in consistency on prolonged storage

To avoid this rheological studies must be performed. Slight change in temperature may affect the consistency of the product. Therefore they must be stored at controlled temperatures.

3. Oxidation

Ointment bases like wool fat and wool alcohol are liable to undergo oxidation reactions and antioxidants are to be added in such preparations.

4. Hydrolysis

Drugs susceptible to hydrolysis must be dispensed in an anhydrous base to avoid hydrolytic degradation.

Pastes

Pastes are semi-solid preparations meant for external application to skin. They are stiff in nature, and do not melt at ordinary temperature and thus form a protective coating over the areas to which they are applied. Ointments and pastes can be differentiated as follows :

Pastes	Ointments
Pastes are concentrates of absorptive powders dispersed in hydrophillic petrolatum.	Ointments are semi-solid preparations meant for external application to the skin or mucous membrane.
They contain large amount of finely powdered solids such as starch, ZnO, CaCO$_3$.	They contain medicament dissolved/suspended/emulsified in the base. They are soft semi- solid preparations.

Contd.

Pastes	Ointments
They are less greasy.	They are more greasy.
They are less macerating than ointments.	They are more macerating in action.
Pastes contain large amount of powder which is porous in nature hence perspiration can escape.	They are used for the protection of lesions.
They are applied generously either with a spatula or spread on lint.	Use of spatula is not necessary.

Classification of pastes

Pastes can be classified according to the type of ointment base used. Some examples with their uses are given in the following table.

Table 7.3.

Name of base	Examples	Uses
1. Hydrocarbon base	(a) Soft paraffin for compound zinc paste B.P. and compound zinc and salicylic acid paste B.P. (Lassar's paste)	For treatment of eczema, psoriasis.
	(b) Liquid paraffin for compound aluminium paste (Baltimore paste B.P.C.)	To protect skin from the discharge of colostomies, leostomies.
2. Water miscible base	(a) Emulsifying ointment for resorcinol and sulphur paste B.P.C.	For treatment of dandruff.
	(b) Magnesium sulphate paste (Morison's paste) B.P.C. containing dry magnesium sulphate (45% w/w), phenol and glycerin.	For treatment of boils.
	(c) Titanium dioxide paste B.P.C. containing titanium dioxide, zinc oxide, light kaolin, and red ferric oxide in glycerin and water.	Useful for absorbing exudations from weeping skin conditions.

Contd.

Name of base	Examples	Uses
3. Water soluble base	(a) Macrogol bases	Anti-inflammatory.
	(b) Triamcinolone dental paste B.P.C. is a dispersion of triamcinolone acetonide in an adhesive paste.,	

Preparation of pastes

1. Fusion method (semi-solid base)

Example : Zinc and coal tar paste B.P.C.

Formula :

Zinc oxide, fine form

Coal tar

Emulsifying wax

Starch

Yellow soft paraffin

Procedure

1. Melt the required amount of wax in a tared dish at a temperature not more than 70°C.
2. Mix it with weighed amount of coal tar.
3. Melt the soft paraffin in a separate dish but temperature should not exceed 70°C. Add about half of the melted soft paraffin to tar and wax mixture.
4. Mix it well. Add the remainder of paraffin. Stir it again to get a homogenous product.
5. Allow it to cool to about 30°C and add zinc oxide (passed through sieve No. 180), stir slowly with continuous stirring.
6. Pack in a well-closed container.

2. Trituration method (liquid vehicle)

Example : Magnesium sulphate paste B.P.C. (Morison's paste)

Dry magnesium sulphate (dried at 150°C and cooled)

Phenol

Glycerol (heated to 120°C and cooled)

Procedure

1. Dissolve the phenol in glycerol.
2. Put the dried magnesium sulphate in a warm dry mortar and levigate, with gradually increasing volumes of the solution.
3. Pack in a well-closed jar.

Note : This paste should be free from micro-organisms because it is used to draw out contents of boils and hence it should not cause re-infection.

3. Combination of fusion and trituration method

Example : Compound zinc paste or semi-solid base
Formula :

Zinc oxide, finely sifted

Starch

White soft paraffin

Procedure

1. Melt the base at a low temperature and pass the powder through sieve No. 180.
2. Mix the base thoroughly with weighed amount of powder in a warm mortar to get a smooth, homogenous product. Cool it.
3. Pack it in a well-closed container.

Jellies

Definition

Jellies are transparent or translucent, non-greasy, semi-solid gels generally meant for external application. They are used for medication, lubrication and some miscellaneous applications.

1. Medicated jellies

As jellies contain sufficient water, therefore they are suitable for water soluble medicaments such as local anaesthetics, antiseptics, etc. After evaporation of water, jellies provide a local cooling effect and the residual film gives protection. Few examples of medicated jellies are represented here.

(i) Ephedrine sulphate is used as a vasoconstrictor to arrest the bleeding of nose.
(ii) Phenyl mercuric nitrate is used as a spermicidal contraceptive.

2. Lubricants

Jellies are used for lubrication of diagnostic equipments such as rubber gloves, cystoscopes, fingerstalls, etc. For this a thin, transparent, water soluble, lubricant jelly should be used. It should be sterile.

3. Miscellaneous jellies

They serve the following purposes :

(a) *Patch testing*

Here jellies are used as a vehicle for allergens which is applied to the skin to check the sensitivity. After drying, it leaves a residual film which helps to keep the patches separate.

(b) *Electrocardiography*

Electrode jelly is used to reduce the electrical resistance between the patient's skin and the electrode. This jelly contains NaCl (which is a good conductor), pumice powder and glycerol (humectant).

Table 7.4. Preparation of different jellies

Type of preparation		Formula	Method of preparation
I.	Tragacanth jelly	Ichthammol, tragacanth, alcohol (90%), glycerin, water	1. Prepare tragacanth mucilage in a wide-mouth jar. 2. Mix ichthammol and glycerin with small quantity of water. Add to the mucilage and shake well. 3. Add remaining water to make up the final volume and reshake. 4. Pack it in a internally lacquered aluminium tube.
II.	Jelly base made with sodium alginate	Sodium alginate, glycerin, methyl hydroxy benzoate, calcium gluconates, water	1. Wet the sodium alginate with glycerin in a glass mortar. 2. Dissolve the preservative and calcium gluconate in about 3/4th of water with the help of heat. Cool to about 60°C and stir it well. 3. Add sodium alginate glycerin mixture to it in small amounts and stir it vigorously. 4. Pack it in a well-closed container.

Contd.

Type of preparation	Formula	Method of preparation
III. Jelly with a gelatinised starch base	Resorcinol, ichthammol, starch glycerin (B.P.C. 1963)	Finely powder resorcinol and mix it with little of starch glycerin on a tile. Add ichthammol to it. Mix it well. Add remaining quantity of base to make the final preparation. Pack it in a well-closed container.
IV. Glycero-gelatin jelly	Zinc oxide, gelatin, glycerol, water	1. Finely powder zinc oxide and pass it through sieve No. 180. Add zinc oxide to molten glycero-gelatin base with continuous stirring. 2. Pour it into a tray and keep it aside for some time. Cut into pieces with a sharp razor or knife.
V. Lubricating jelly with a cellulose ether base	Sodium carboxy methyl cellulose, glycerol, methyl hydroxy benzoate, patent blue V (dye), water	1. Dissolve methyl hydroxy benzoate in water using heat. 2. Mix sodium carboxy methyl cellulose with glycerin in a glass mortar. 3. Pour this mixture into methyl hydroxy benzoate solution. 4. Stir it well until a clear gel is formed. Add dye solution to it. Make up the volume. Pack it in a tube.
VI. Carbomer jelly	Ephedrine sulphate, carbopol triethanolamine, water	1. Dissolve ephedrine sulphate in 3/4th of water. 2. Add carbopol to it with vigorous stirring until a lump-free dispersion is obtained. 3. Add triethanolamine drop by drop with gentle stirring. 4. Add remaining quantity of water to make up the volume.
VII. Bentonite gel	Zinc oxide, glycerol, bentonite, water	Mix zinc oxide in fine form with bentonite in a mortar and triturate with glycerol. Add water in small amount with constant stirring.

Poultice

Poultices are the viscous wet mass of solid substances applied to the skin for their fomentation action in order to give relief from pain or reduce inflammation or to act as a counter-irritant. For use, poultice is first heated and then it is spread thickly on some dressing or cloth and applied to the affected area which is sometimes already covered with muslin to facilitate the removal after use. Generally they are prepared by using clays such as heavy kaolin. A very important example of poultice is kaolin poultice B.P.C.

Formula :

> Heavy kaolin, dried at 100°C and finely sifted
> Thymol
> Boric acid, finely sifted
> Peppermint oil
> Methyl salicylate
> Glycerol

In this glycerol being hygroscopic in nature draws infected material from the tissue. Methyl salicylate is an anti-rheumatic drug. Thymol is a powerful bactericide, boric acid acts as a weak antimicrobial agent. In market, kaolin is generally supplied in tins so that it can withstand heating in water.

Method of preparation

1. Mix finely sifted boric acid and heavy kaolin (dried and sifted) in a mortar. Gradually triturate it with glycerol to form a smooth paste.
2. Transfer it to a heat-resistant glass container and heat it at 120°C for 1 hr. in a hot air oven with occasional stirring.
3. Cool it, add the remaining ingredients to it with vigorous stirring.
4. Pack it in a close container to prevent absorption of moisture.

8

Suppositories and Pessaries

Suppositories are medicated solid dosage forms of special shape meant for insertion into body cavities other than oral cavity. They may be inserted into rectum, vagina or nasal cavity. Those intended for vagina are called pessaries. The medicament is incorporated into base such as cocoa butter which melts at body temperature to release the medicament.

Suppositories are particularly meant for local action, systemic action and for mechanical action.

Advantages of suppositories

Suppositories have the following advantages :

1. They can be easily administered to children and old persons.
2. It is a unit solid dosage form.
3. Whenever local effect is required, it can be placed directly at the site of action.
4. They may be used for treating patients who are unconscious or mentally disturbed.
5. They can be used conveniently for medicaments which cannot be given orally for the following reasons :

    (a) drugs which irritate gastro-intestinal tract;
    (b) drugs which cause vomitting;
    (c) drugs which are destroyed by stomach pH or undergo hepatic first pass metabolism.

6. Rapid action of drug is produced because rectum provides a good absorption surface area from which soluble substances can pass quickly.

Disadvantages

The major and only disadvantage of suppositories is the aesthetic objection to the patient while introducing a sold mass into a body cavity.

Types of Suppositories

1. Rectal suppositories

These are meant for introduction into the rectum for their systemic effect. They are generally made up of theobroma oil and weigh 1-2 g. They are tapered at one or both ends. Rectal suppositories vary in sizes to meet the needs of infants, children and adults. Those meant for children are smaller in size and weigh about 1 g.

2. Vaginal suppositories or pessaries

Pessaries differ from rectal suppositories in their size, shape and weight. Vaginal suppositories may be conical, rod-shaped, or wedge-shaped. Their weight varies from 4 g to 8 g. They are meant for local action on vagina. Nowadays vaginal capsules and tablets are also available.

3. Urethral suppositories or urethral bougies

These are thin, long, cylindrical forms rounded at one end to facilitate insertion. Their weight varies from 2 g to 4 g.

Sex	Diameter	Length	Weight
Female	3-6 mm	70 mm	2 gm
Male	3-6 mm	140 mm	4 gm

4. Nasal suppositories or nasal bougies or bouginaria

These are meant for introduction into the nasal cavity and are similar to urethral suppositories. They are about 9-10 cm long and weigh about 1 g. Glycero-gelatin base is used for the preparation of nasal suppositories.

5. Ear cones or aurinaria

Nowadays these are rarely used. Generally theobroma oil is used as a base.

Suppository Bases

Suppository bases are of three types :

1. Oily bases
2. Water miscible and water soluble bases
3. Synthetic bases

Characteristics of an ideal base :

1. It should melt at body temperature or dissolve in body fluids.

2. It should be stable if heated above its melting point.
3. It should release the medicament readily.
4. It should be non-toxic and non-irritant.
5. It should be compatible with large number of drugs.
6. It should not stick to side of mould and should be easily mouldable.
7. It should remain stable on prolonged storage.
8. It should be good in appearance.

1. Oily bases

(a) *Theobroma oil or cocoa butter*

It is a yellowish white solid obtained from crushed and roasted seeds of theobroma cocoa.

Properties

(a) M.P. — 30-35°C.
(b) Consistency — butter-like.
(c) Odour — chocolate-like.
(d) Composition — mixture of glyceryl esters of stearic, palmitic, oleic and other fatty acids.
(e) This base melts at body temperature and releases the medicament for rapid absorption. Cocoa butter is suitable for rectal suppositories but not for pessaries, bouginaria and urethral bougies because of its immiscibility with mucous secretions.

Disadvantages

(a) Polymorphism : It shows the phenomenon of polymorphism, i.e., when melted and cooled theobroma oil solidifies into different crystalline forms depending upon melting temperature, rate of cooling and size of mass.

Temperature of melting	After cooling
At 20°C	Alpha crystals
Not more than 36°C	Slow cooling forms stable beta crystals
Overheating	Unstable gamma crystals*

* These unstable forms return to stable form after several days.

(b) It has a tendency to stick to the sides of moulds when solidified.
(c) It becomes rancid and melts in warm weather.

(d) Sometimes melted base may escape from the rectum or vagina, i.e., leakage from body cavities can take place.

(e) It is immiscible with body fluids.

(f) Relatively cost is high.

(g) When certain drugs are added to cocoa butter liquefaction takes place, e.g., chloral hydrate, lactic acid. Bees wax can be added to maintain the consistency in such cases.

(b) *Emulsified theobroma oil*

This may be used as a base when large quantities of aqueous solutions are to be incorporated. To prepare suppositories using emulsified theobroma oil as a base, we can add 5% glyceryl monostearate, 10% lanette wax, 2-3% cetyl alcohol, 4% bees wax and 12% spermaceti.

(c) *Hydrogenated oils*

These are obtained by hydrogenation and subsequent heat treatment of vegetable oils such as arachis oil, cotton seed oil. Hydrogenation saturates unsaturated glycerides. It is used as a substitute for theobroma oil.

2. Water miscible or water soluble bases

(a) *Glycero-gelatin bases*

It is a mixture of glycerin and water which is made into a stiff jelly by the addition of gelatin. This base is used for making jellies, pessaries and suppositories.

These suppositories are translucent gelatinous solids which tend to dissolve or disperse slowly in the body cavity and release the medicament. Hence they are preferred over fatty bases. Glycero-gelatin base is well suited for suppositories containing boric acid, chloral hydrate, bromides, iodides, opium, etc.

To avoid incompatible reactions, suitable type of gelatin is used. Two grades of gelatin are available :

1. Pharmagel A (Type A) — acidic in nature and used for acidic drugs; iso-electric point (7-9).

2. Pharmagel B (Type B) — alkaline in nature and used for alkaline drugs; iso-electric point (4.7-5).

Formulae of few common bases

(i) Mass of glycerin suppositories B.P.

   Gelatin   14% w/w

   (percentage of gelatin can be varied up to 25%)

Glycerol   70% w/w
(according to the requirement)
(ii) Gelato-glycerol B.P.C.
Gelatin   32.5 %
Glycerol   40   %

Disadvantages

1. They are hygroscopic in nature therefore they must be stored well.
2. Their solution time depends upon the content and quality of gelatin used.
3. They are more difficult to prepare and handle.
4. They have a physiological action (laxative).
5. Gelatin is incompatible with protein components, e.g., tannic acid.
6. Suitable preservation is required as chances of bacterial growth and mould growth are frequent.

(b) *Soap glycerin suppositories*

Soap replaces gelatin from glycero-gelatin bases which make the glycerin sufficiently stiff to prepare a suppository and further soap helps in the evacuation action of glycerin. The only disadvantage is that they are very hygroscopic and therefore should be protected from atmospheric moisture.

(c) *Polyethylene glycols*

Polyethylene glycol polymers are commonly known as carbowaxes or polyglycols or macrogols. Their physical form varies according to their mol. wt.

Mol. wt.	Physical form
Macrogol (less than 1000)	Liquids
Macrogol (more than 1000)	Waxy solids

Advantages

(i) They are non-irritant and chemically stable.
(ii) Physical properties can be varied by the addition of high and low mol. wt. polymers.
(iii) They provide prolonged action because they do not melt in the body cavity (high M.P.) but dissolve slowly for a long time.

(iv) Macrogols do not stick to the side of mould.

(v) They absorb water well and have excellent solvent properties.

(vi) Suppositories made from macrogols have clean and smooth appearance.

Disadvantages

(i) They are hygroscopic and hence require special storage containers.

(ii) They are incompatible with certain drugs like tannins, phenols, etc.

(iii) High solubility of macrogols leads to supersaturation which in turn makes crystals and fracture the product on storage.

(iv) Their good solvent property can result in retention of the drug in the liquefied base, thereby reducing their therapeutic activity.

3. Synthetic bases

Advantages over theobroma oil

(i) Lubrication of mould is not required.

(ii) Overheating does not affect the solidifying points.

(iii) They solidify rapidly.

(iv) Their emulsifying and water absorbing capacities are good.

(v) Non-irritant.

(vi) White, odourless, clean and attractive suppositories are produced.

(vii) They are resistant to oxidation.

Disadvantages

(i) They should not be cooled rapidly in a refrigerator because they become brittle.

(ii) They are less viscous on melting which results in sedimentation of other substances.

A number of proprietary synthetic bases are available.

(a) **Massa estarinum.** It consists of a mixture of mono-, di- and triglycerides of saturated fatty acids of formula $C_{11}H_{23}COOH$ to $C_{17}H_{35}COOH$. They are odourless, colourless, brittle solids. Several grades are available but generally grade B is recommended. It has a melting point 33.5-35.5°C.

(b) **Witespol.** They consist of triglycerides of saturated vegetable acids (chain length C_{12}—C_{18}) with varying percentage of partial esters. Nine grades are available.

(c) **Massuppol.** This consists of glyceryl esters, mainly of lauric acid to which small amount of glyceryl monostearate has been added to increase water absorption capacity.

Preparation of suppositories

Generally suppositories and pessaries are prepared in dispensaries using metallic moulds having six or twelve cavities. They can be opened for lubrication by removing a screw. For cleaning the opened plates are immersed in hot water containing a detergent. Then they are wiped gently with a soft cloth and dried thoroughly. The nominal capacities of the common moulds are 1 g (15 gr), 2 g (30 gr), 4 g (60 gr) and 8 g (120 gr).

Calibration of mould

Generally a standard mould of 15 grain or 1 g capacity is used. Calibration of mould is necessary for all moulds because the size of suppository from a particular mould remains same but the weight varies. This is due to density of different medicaments and bases. This is done by making use of displacement values. It is defined as "The quantity of drug which displaces one part of the base". Displacement values of few medicaments in suppositories using cocoa butter as a base are listed below.

Table 8.1.

Name of medicament	Displacement value
Aminophylline	1.5
Boric acid	1.5
Bismuth subgallate	3.0
Castor oil	1.0
Chloral hydrate	1.5
Cocaine hydrochloride	1.5
Hammelis dry extract	1.5
Hydrocortisone acetate	1.5
Ichthammol	1.0
Iodoform	4.0
Liquids	1.0
Morphine hydrochloride	1.5
Peru balsam	1.0
Phenobarbitone	1.0
Resorcinol	1.0
Tannic acid	1.0
Zinc oxide	5.0

Calculation of displacement value

Displacement value of a medicament can be calculated as follows :

1. Prepare and weigh 8 suppositories containing theobroma oil (or other base) = a g.
2. Prepare and weigh 8 suppositories containing 40% medicament = b g.
3. Calculate the amount of theobroma oil present in 8 medicated suppositories = c g.
4. Calculate the amount of medicament present in medicated suppositories = d g.
5. Calculate the amount of theobroma oil displaced by d g of medicament. Let it be $a - c$ g.

$$\text{Displacement value of medicament} = \frac{d}{a - c}$$

Example : Calculate the displacement value of zinc oxide in a suppository using cocoa butter as a base when it contains 40% of medicament and is prepared in 1 g mould. The weight of 8 suppositories is 11.74 g.

Solution :

(a) Weight of 8 suppositories containing theobroma oil alone = 1×8
    = 8 g   (mould size is 1 g)

(b) Weight of 8 suppositories containing 40% medicament = 11.74 g.

(c) Amount of theobroma oil present = $\dfrac{60}{100} \times 11.74 = 7.044$ g.

(d) Amount of medicament present = $\dfrac{40}{100} \times 11.74 = 4.696$ g.

(e) Amount of theobroma oil displaced by 4.696 g of medicament = 8 – 7.044 = 0.956 g.

$$\text{Displacement value} = \frac{4.696}{0.956} = 4.912 \text{ (approx. 5)}$$

Lubrication of mould

Lubrication is necessary for glycero-gelatin base or for cocoa butter because of their sticky nature. The lubricant must be of different nature from the suppository base to provide a buffer film between the suppository and the metal of the mould. Hence an oily lubricant is used for glycero-gelatin suppositories and aqueous lubricant is used for cocoa butter suppositories.

For cocoa butter suppositories

Soft soap 10 g

Glycerol 10 ml

Alcohol (90%) 50 ml

For glycero-gelatin suppositories

Liquid paraffin or arachis oil

It is not necessary to lubricate the mould when synthetic bases or macrogol bases are used.

For lubrication, the lubricant should be applied on a pad of gauze or a muslin cloth or with the help of a soft brush. Cotton wool should never be used because it shreds fibres. After lubrication, the mould should be closed and kept on white tile to drain the excess.

Methods of preparation

1. Fusion method
2. Compression method

1. Fusion method

(i) Thoroughly clean and lubricate the mould and invert it on ice to drain and cool.

(ii) Heat the dish over water bath, to this add weighed amount of base. Remove the dish when two thirds of the base melts. This will prevent overheating of the base.

(iii) Place the weighed quantity of medicament on a warmed tile. Over it pour about half the melted base. Mix it thoroughly with a flexible spatula and transfer the mixed mass to a dish and stir to form a homogenous mass. Warm the dish over water bath for few seconds so that the mass becomes pourable.

(iv) Pour this melted mass into the cavities of mould kept over ice. Fill each cavity to overflowing to prevent the formation of hollow voids on cooling. Precaution must be taken while filling the cavities to stir continuously to ensure even distribution of medicament.

(v) When the mass just sets, remove the excess of mass with a sharp knife or blade.

(vi) Keep the mould in a cool place or over ice for 10-15 minutes.

(vii) Open the mould, and remove the suppositories.

2. Compression method

As this method does not require heat so it is best suitable for the thermolabile and insoluble drugs. It is unsuitable for glvcero-gelatin suppositories and is of little value where melting is essential for the preparation of mass.

Method

(i) Thoroughly mix the powdered medicament with an equal amount of cocoa butter in a mortar.

(ii) Then add remaining quantity of grated cocoa butter gradually. Allowance is made for unavoidable wastage.

(iii) Mixed mass is forced into the cavities of mould by applying pressure to the handle of machine.

(iv) The pressure is further applied, stop plate is removed and finished suppositories are obtained.

On large scale manufacturing the hydraulically operated cold-compression machines are used.

Use of suppositories for drug absorption

Suppositories are particularly useful when the drug cannot be taken orally or the drug is liable to be destroyed by the liver. Drugs are absorbed by rectal route through rich blood supply in anorectal region. By this route, drugs are rapidly absorbed and get quickly distributed into circulation which bypasses the liver. It also provides neutral pH which is very advantageous to stability of many drugs. For complete therapeutic effect, the drug used in suppository must be

(i) in very fine state of subdivision;

(ii) uniformly distributed in base;

(iii) in a readily absorbable form.

The effectiveness of suppository also depends upon the rate of diffusion of the drug from the base to the surrounding.

Packaging of suppositories

Generally suppositories are packaged in partition boxes which can hold them in upright position. Many commercial suppositories are wrapped separately in aluminum foil or PVC-polyethylene strip. Glycerin and glycero-gelatin suppositories are often packed in tightly closed screw-capped glass containers. For large scale manufacturing, nowadays suppositories are directly moulded into its primary packaging which consists of plastic material or aluminum foils. The moulds are sealed and excess is then trimmed off and packed in cartons.

9

Dental and Cosmetic Preparations

The word cosmetic is defined by 'cosmos' meaning universe which refers particularly to the 'effect of sun rays on skin'. This can be prevented by use of cosmetics. Skin not only covers the body but performs various protective and regulatory functions to maintain the integrity of individual. Cosmetics serve one of the following functions :

 (i) Avoid premature ageing of skin.

 (ii) Give a sense of well-being.

 (iii) Maintain body health and hygiene.

 (iv) Improve overall looks and personality.

 Cosmetic preparations include cleansing lotions, creams, skin tonics, antidandruff preparations, hair dyes, lipsticks, deodorants, etc., whereas dentifrices include tooth powders and tooth pastes.

Dental Preparations

Dentifrices are the preparations meant for removal of food debris from tooth cavity. Food debris is responsible for the growth of bacteria which in turn leads to decalcification of tooth enamel and the formation of cavities. They are presented in following forms :

 (i) Tooth powders

 (ii) Tooth pastes

 (iii) Liquid preparations.

 The teeth are hard, calcified structures firmly present in bony sockets of upper and lower jaws. Dentifrices perform the following functions :

 (i) Cleansing of tooth

 (ii) Tooth root polishing

 (iii) Removal of stains

 (iv) Reduce incidence of tooth decay

 (v) Reduction of mouth odours.

Tooth powders include abrasive substances, surface active detergents, flavouring oils, and sweetening agents. Along with above mentioned ingredients tooth pastes include water, humectant, binder and a preservative.

Abrasives are added for polishing and cleaning of teeth, e.g., calcium carbonate, calcium phosphate, dicalcium phosphate dihydrate, calcium pyrophosphate, etc. A detergent is added along with abrasives to lower the surface tension and loosen the surface deposit. The detergent must be non-toxic and non-irritant, e.g., sodium lauryl sulphate, sodium N-lauryl sarcosinate, sodium alkyl sulfosuccinate, etc. Humectants are added in a paste to retain moisture. It helps in producing a paste that will remain mobile even if the cap is not firmly closed, e.g., glycerol, propylene glycol, sorbitol, etc. Binding agents prevent separation of solid and liquid phases during storage. Mainly they are cellulose derivatives, e.g., sodium alginate, tragacanth, gum arabic and gum karaya, etc. Colouring agents and flavouring agents are added to make the product popular and acceptable to the people. Flavours which are generally used are peppermint, spearmint, wintergreen and cinnamon-mint.

Method of preparation

Tooth powders are prepared in big blending and mixing tanks. All the solid ingredients are weighed and mixed thoroughly in ascending order of their weights. Flavouring agents can be sprayed over powder particles during mixing process. Then they are packed in metallic/plastic sifter-top containers.

For tooth pastes, equipment used should be of stainless steel or glass-lined type. Mixture of binder and humectant is dispersed in a liquid containing saccharin and preservative. It is then allowed to swell to form a homogenous even gel. This gel is then pumped into suitable mixing tank. Abrasives are added slowly with agitation until a uniform paste is formed. To this are added flavouring agent and detergent with thorough distribution. They are finally packed in collapsible tubes.

Formulae :

1. Precipitated calcium carbonate   95%
    Sodium palmitate   5%
    Flavouring and sweetening agent q.s.

2. Dicalcium phosphate dihydrate   79%
    Precipitated calcium carbonate   20%
    Sodium lauryl sulphate   1%
    Flavouring and sweetening agent q.s.

Facial Cosmetics

Facial cosmetics are used for cleansing, refreshing and nourishing effects. They are available in solid, liquid, and semi-solid dosage forms. A large variety of facial cosmetics are available to preserve health and suppleness of facial skin. They prevent premature ageing of skin and improve the overall looks and personality.

Facial cosmetics include :

1. Face powders
2. Cleansing creams and cleansing lotions
3. Cold creams
4. Foundation creams
5. Vanishing creams
6. Moisturising creams
7. Skin tonics
8. Lipsticks
9. Shaving creams
10. After shave preparations.

Face Powders

Face powder is a cosmetic preparation meant for improvement of overall attractiveness of the face. It provides a visual covering to skin and imparts smooth finish to it.

Face powders are available in a variety of colour shades. The most important property is its uniform spreadability. Since there is no single ingredient that possesses all the properties desired in a face powder, a blend of ingredients is used.

Face powders generally contain talcum powder, kaolin, precipitated chalk, magnesium carbonate, zinc oxide, titanium dioxide, starch, etc. Titanium dioxide acts as an opacifying agent while magnesium carbonate has absorbent properties. Kaolin provides soothing effect to the skin.

Compact face powder is a dry powder which has been compressed to form a cake and is usually applied with powder puff. Suitable binding agents are added to the above mentioned formula to bind the powder particles, e.g., magnesium stearates, polyvinyl pyrollidone, methyl cellulose, etc.

Formulae :

1.	Talcum	75%
	Kaolin	5%
	Chalk precipitated	5%

Zinc stearate	5%
Zinc oxide	10%
Perfume and colour q.s.	
2. Talcum	60%
Titanium dioxide	5%
Zinc oxide	15%
Chalk precipitated	13%
Zinc stearate	7%
Perfume and colour q.s.	

Cleansing Creams and Cleansing Lotions

Cleansing creams

Cleansing creams are used to remove facial make-up. These creams form an emollient film on the skin which is protective in a dry skin condition. They are basically cold creams and consist of a detergent for cleansing action and further ingredients may be added to soften, lubricate and protect the skin. Cleansing creams require oils to dissolve unwanted materials on the skin. This oily phase may be of olive oil, expressed almond oil or liquid paraffin. For o/w type cleansing creams tweens are used along with detergent for removal of dirt. Triethanolamine, sodium lauryl sulphate can also be added. Sodium lauryl sulphate, and alkyl sulphate provide stability to the preparation along with its detergent action. Pepsin is sometimes added to make facial skin smooth.

There are three types of cleansing creams :

1. Bees wax — borax emulsion type
2. Liquefying type
3. Miscellaneous emulsion type
   (a) Sorbitan fatty acid ester emulsion creams
   (b) Creams prepared from glycerol, sodium cetyl sulphate, etc.
   (c) Acid containing cleansing creams
   (d) Detergent cleansing creams
   (e) Antibacterial cleansing creams

Formulae :

1. Bees wax	16.67	%
Mineral oil	50	%
Borax	0.83	%
Water	32.5	%
Perfume q.s.		

2. Stearic acid   16   %
   Potassium hydroxide   0.8   %
   P.E.G. monostearate   10   %
   Glycerol   5   %
   Water   68   %
   Preservative   0.2   %

Cleansing lotions

Cleansing lotions are used as alternatives to cleansing creams and they are more convenient to use during daytime. They contain less oily material than cleansing creams and do not leave a residual film of oil on the skin after use.

Two types of cleansing lotions are used :

(i) Solution type

(ii) Emulsion type (o/w)

Emulsion type cleansing lotions generally contain triethanolamine stearate, glyceryl monostearate, fatty alcohols, stearic acid, bees wax and mineral oil, etc. Triethanolamine acts as an emulsifying agent while glyceryl monostearate, stearic acid, fatty alcohols are used to increase stability and thickness of the preparation.

Formulae :

1. Triethanolamine stearate   8%
   Mineral oil   35%
   Bees wax   8%
   Water   55%

2. Ethanol   10   %
   Menthol   0.75   %
   Camphor   0.2   %
   Hexachlorophene   0.1   %
   Cetyl alcohol   2   %
   Stearyl amine   2   %
   Water up to   100   %

Cold Creams

Cold cream is an emulsion in which the proportion of fatty and oily materials are mixed and when it is applied to the skin a cooling effect is produced due to slow evaporation of water present in the emulsion.

Earlier cold creams consisted of animal and vegetable fats. As vegetable oils have tendency to get rancid, they are replaced by mineral oil which gives a more stable product. Physically these creams are o/w type emulsions but after application on skin, sufficient water evaporates to permit phase inversion to w/o type, with the oil as external phase.

USP formula consists of the following ingredients :

Emulsifying wax	125	gm
White bees wax	120	gm
Liquid paraffin	560	gm
Sodium borate	5	gm
Rose water	25	ml
Rose oil	0.2	ml
Purified water	165	ml

Method of preparation

1. Waxes and oil are melted by heating to 70°C. Separately dissolve sodium borate in rose water and water. Heat it to 70°C.
2. Slowly add the aqueous phase containing sodium borate to oily phase with continuous stirring until it has cooled down to about 45°C.
3. To this add required amount of rose oil and stir it well until the product is just pourable.
4. Pack it, label and dispense it as directed.

Foundation Creams

Foundation creams are used to provide a smooth emollient base for application of facial make-up. They also act as skin protectives to prevent the damage caused by environmental factors like sun or wind.

Ideal properties of foundation creams

1. It should provide a non-greasy and non-occlusive film on the face.
2. It should improve the adhesion of face powder for a longer period of time.
3. It should remain stable and should not damage the skin.
4. It should have suitable thixotropic consistency.

Originally foundation creams were known as vanishing creams which were applied before the application of powder. Foundation creams are invariably based on o/w systems, although w/o preparations are available for dry skin.

Foundation creams contain fatty materials, stearic acid, alkalies, glycerin, surfactants, emulsifying agents, pigments, preservatives and perfumes, etc. Fatty materials like bees wax, carnauba wax, lanolin and mineral oil are used to provide emollient effect. Sodium hydroxide is preferred over potassium hydroxide and certain ionic and non-ionic surfactants are added for emulsification. Titanium dioxide is used to impart more dark and intense colour to the skin. It also covers the skin blemishes and other skin marks. Preservatives like benzoic acid (0.2%), and salicylic acid (0.2%) are added to these preparations.

Liquid foundation creams are often designated as 'beauty milks'. Since these preparations contain large proportion of water, they are liable to lose some of it by evaporation. Therefore the product should be packed in an airtight container with a narrow neck.

Formulae : O/w emulsion type

Part A

Stearic acid	15	%
Span 60	2.5	%
Isopropyl palmitate	2	%

Part B

Tween 60	1.5	%
Propylene glycol	10	%
Water	54	%
Dry powders (titanium dioxide, talcum, inorganic pigments)	15	%
Preservative q.s.		
Perfume q.s.		

Heat the above mentioned ingredients of Part A to 85°C and B to 90°C in separate containers. Add B to A and agitate while cooling. Perfume is added after cooling it to a temperature of 45°C and packed.

Vanishing Creams

Vanishing creams when applied to the skin leave an almost invisible layer on it and hence they are named vanishing creams. These creams can be quickly washed off with water due to presence of o/w emulsifiers.

Formula of vanishing creams includes oil, stearic acid, alkali and water. A good vanishing cream always gives a pearly white shining product, which on application gives a thin white film of free stearic acid. Perfumes like vanillin, eugenol, etc., must be added to it.

Although this formula seems to be very simple but it is very difficult to prepare vanishing creams because of variation in composition of commercial stearic acid known as 'stearin'. This stearin is a mixture of palmitic and stearic acid together with a small quantity of oleic acid.

Vanishing creams may lose some of their water by evaporation forming an unstable product therefore they should be packed in airtight containers.

Formulae :

1. Stearic acid   15.30 %
   Potassium hydroxide   0.7 %
   Glycerine   8 %
   Water   76.3 %
   Preservative and perfume q.s.
2. Stearic acid   17 %
   Glyceryl monostearate   1 %
   Cetyl alcohol   1 %
   Glycerine   6 %
   Caustic potash (100%)   0.75 %
   Caustic soda (100%)   0.25 %
   Distilled water   74 %
   Preservative and perfume q.s.

Moisturising Creams

A dry skin condition cannot be corrected by fatty creams alone because they only prevent water loss by evaporation. Secondly these creams are applied at night. During day time their application is not useful. Moisturising creams serve following purposes :

1. It gives protection to skin against bacteria.
2. It gives fresher and natural appearance to the skin.
3. They help to preserve the skin in a soft, supple condition.
4. They maintain moisture content and prevent a dry condition.

Moisturising creams contain materials like humectants (glycerin, sorbitol, propylene glycol, lipophillic substances, mineral oil, vegetable oil, lanolin, etc.) and water. Moisturising preparations can be either in cream or lotion form. They are used on the skin before applying make-up.

Skin Tonics

Skin tonics or face tonics are used for cleansing and care of facial skin. These preparations provide cooling and refreshing effects, therefore they are called 'skin freshner' or 'toning lotions'. The usual skin tonics contain some alcohol having a slight astringent effect, but a high alcohol content may cause stinging effect. Besides alcohol, glycerin is added to prevent dryness. Surfactants are also sometimes added to increase cleansing action and to solubilise perfumes. Most cleansers remove the skin acidity but the tonics immediately restore proper acid balance. Some of the formulae are mentioned below.

Formulae :

1. Alcohol   20   %
   Orange flower water   30   %
   Rose water   30   %
   Potassium aluminium sulphate   0.5 %
   Water   19.5 %
   Preservative q.s.

2. Zinc phenol sulphonate   1%
   Glycerine   10%
   Camphor water   20%
   Alcohol   10%
   Rose water   40%
   Water   19%
   Preservative q.s.

Some hormonal and non-hormonal compounds are also used as skin tonics. Hormones like estrogens having water holding capacity provide a feeling of fullness to the skin. Similarly non-hormonal compounds like pregnenolone 0.5% counteract wrinkles by causing hydration and plumping of the skin.

Pre-shave and After-shave Preparations

Under less favourable conditions shaving generally leads to discomfort, irritation and actual damage to the skin. This can be reduced by using a shaving product which can prepare the face adequately for shaving, allow a comfortable, painless shave and leave a refreshing effect after the shave is over.

Pre-shave preparations

Pre-shave preparations are used for the following purposes :

   (i)   To prepare the beard and skin of the face.
   (ii) To increase lubricity.
   (iii) To soften the hair.
   (iv) To reduce sensitivity of skin to mechanical and chemical effects of shaving.

1. Shaving soaps

Shaving soaps are prepared in cake form and are applied with the help of shaving brush to produce a sufficient quantity of lather. Coconut oil soaps produce thick lather quickly. Formula includes tallow, coconut oil, stearic acid, sodium hydroxide and potassium hydroxide. They are prepared by melting method.

2. Shaving sticks

Shaving sticks are usually produced in a very dry form which is rubbed onto the moistened skin, then lather is produced with the help of brush. Shaving sticks generally comprise of stearic acid, coconut oil, potassium hydroxide, sodium hydroxide and glycerol.

3. Lather shaving creams

Lather shaving creams contain ingredients similar to those present in shaving soap but large quantity of water is present in those creams. Similarly sodium soaps produce a very firm cream while potassium gives a soft and better lathering cream.

Lather shaving creams include stearic acid, coconut oil or fatty acid, glycerol, sodium hydroxide, potassium hydroxide, vegetable or mineral oil and water. They are prepared by saponification of stearic acid using melting method.

4. Non-lathering or brushless shaving creams

They have high lubricating power but cannot soften the beard themselves rapidly. For these creams face has to be first washed with soap and warm water. These creams consist of modified stearate soaps, small proportion of oil, humectants, waxes, emollients and surfactants, etç.

5. Pre-electric-shave preparations

Pre-shave preparations having specialised purposes and functions, can be performed by using talcum powder to absorb moisture and provide a slippery face. This being an alcoholic lotion dries and tautens the skin by its astringent effect. Generally pilomotor active compound is used to erect the beard hair.

After-shave preparations

After-shave preparations are used to relieve the discomfort caused by shaving and to provide cooling, antiseptic and refreshing action. After-shave preparations are available in following dosage forms :

1. Clear lotions

2. Stic-lotions and gels
3. Creams and emulsified lotions
4. Powders
5. Styptics
6. Aerosols

They are prepared by different methods but generally they contain perfume (lavender, sandal wood, eau de cologne), ethanol, menthol, boric acid, lactic acid, aluminium chlorohydrate, humectants (glycerol, sorbitol, propylene glycol), and antiseptics (benzalkonium chloride, cetyl trimethyl ammonium bromide). Menthol provides cooling effect whereas acids help in neutralisation of alkali imparted by soaps. Humectants give emollient effect to the skin.

Formulae :

1. Lather shaving cream

Stearic acid	20-40	%
Coconut oil or fatty acid	6-10	%
Glycerol	5-15	%
ROH	2-6	%
NaOH	1-3	%
Vegetable or mineral oil	1-5	%
Water q.s.		

2. Brushless shaving cream

Stearic acid	10-35	%
Mineral oil	5-15	%
Soap or surfactant	1-3	%
Glycerol	1-10	%
Water	91.5	%

Lipsticks

Lipsticks are used to give an attractive colour and appearance to the lips. Lipsticks can change the apparent facial characteristics and is probably the most frequently used of all the cosmetic products.

Properties of a good lipstick are as follows :

1. It should have an attractive appearance with smooth surface.
2. It should be physically and chemically stable.
3. It should be non-irritant.
4. It should have a good thixotropy.
5. It should provide an appropriate film which could be removed easily.

Formulation of lipsticks

Lipsticks contain following formulation ingredients :

1. Colours
2. Bases
3. Perfumes
4. Antioxidants

Colours used for lipsticks are called bromomixtures due to previous and present use of fluorozine reagent, e.g., eosin (bromo-acid). Other staining dyes are di-bromo fluorescein, (D.C. Orange No. 5), tetrachlorotetrabromo fluorescein (D.C. Red No. 27). Certain pigments are added to intensify the colour, e.g., titanium dioxide. Bases used are mixtures of oils, fatty materials and waxes such as mineral oil, vegetable oil, butyl stearate, cocoa butter, petrolatum, lanolin, lecithin, carnauba wax, bees wax, spermaceti, etc. Perfume selected should be non-irritant and should possess an agreeable taste. Floral, fruity and light spicy fragrances are generally used for this purpose.

Due to oxidation of some ingredients lipsticks get rancid. Therefore it is advisable to use antioxidants like butylated hydroxy anisole, butylated hydroxy toluene, propyl gallate, etc.

Manufacturing of lipsticks involves colour grinding, mixing, molding and flaming.

Formulae :

1.	Carnauba wax	1	%
	Bees wax	15	%
	Lanolin alcohol	5	%
	Cetyl alcohol	5	%
	Castor oil	65	%
	Colouring matter	1-5	%
	Other pigments	5-10	%
	Perfumes	0.5-2	%
2.	Glyceryl monostearate	42	%
	Castor oil	36.8	%
	Mineral oil	8	%
	Pigment	5	%
	Petrolatum	4	%
	Carnauba wax	4	%
	Propyl paraben	0.2	%

Antiperspirants and Deodorants

Antiperspirants are the topical preparations of astringent substances meant for reduction of flow of perspiration. Fresh perspiration of a clean skin has a mild objectionable odour but after some time same perspiration changes considerably due to bacterial decomposition. An effective antiperspirant is therefore designed in such a manner that it should regulate the flow of sweat and prevent the development of odour.

Properties of anti-perspirants are as follows :

1. It should be non-toxic and non-irritant to the skin.
2. It should possess adequate astringent property.
3. It should have no effect on fabrics.
4. It should have a pH 4-4.5 which is very close to normal pH of skin surface.

Several materials having antiperspirant properties have been considered such as aluminium chlorohydrate, an active ingredient having astringent and antibacterial action. Other compounds of aluminium and zinc may be used if they have similar properties and do not cause any irritation to the skin, e.g., aluminium chloride and aluminium sulphate are effective and non-toxic but they cause irritation to skin having an acid reaction with a pH between 2.5-3.0. They may contain stearic acid, mineral oil, bees wax, glyceryl monostearate, etc. Sodium lauryl sulphate, spans and tweens are added to increase the stability of preparation. Titanium dioxide is added in creams to provide a whitening effect.

They are available in various dosage forms like lotions, creams, sprays, powders, etc., having different formulations.

Deodorants

Deodorants are the preparations meant for topical application with suitable antiseptics to arrest or to prevent bacterial decomposition. Deodorants inhibit the bad odour and provide a pleasant one. They are based on bactericidal action.

Formulation of a deodorant preparation includes an antibacterial compound in a suitable base, e.g., zinc oxide (1-15%), boric acid, neomycin, antibiotics, ion exchange resins, and metal chelates, etc.

'Powder' dosage forms are rarely used while 'liquid preparations' are quite effective. They are prepared by dissolving a small amount of antibacterial compound in an aqueous or aqueous-alcoholic lotion containing a light perfume. In both the cases, oil germicide is added. For 'cream deodorants' germicide is added to base vanishing creams (before addition, germicides should be dissolved in sodium hydroxide solution).

Quarternary ammonium compounds require non-ionic medium otherwise they will get inactivated by soaps and other ionic substances.

Efficacy of antiperspirants can be evaluated by following methods :

1. Staining method
2. Gravimetric method
3. Continuously recording method.

Efficacy of deodorants can be tested by an olfactory test of axillary odour. In this test product and control product are applied to axillae of test subjects.

Formulae :

Liquid antiperspirants

Aluminium chlorohydrate	20	%
Propylene glycol	5	%
Alcohol	0.2	%
Perfume q.s.		
Water up to	100	%

Cream antiperspirants

Aluminium chlorohydrate	20%
Glyceryl monostearate (soap free)	20%
Spermaceti	5%
Glycerine	3%
Perfume q.s.	
Water up to	100%

Shampoos

Shampoos can be defined as solid, liquid or semi-solid preparations meant for cleansing action to remove soil and dust from hair without affecting natural gloss of hair.

Properties of shampoos

1. It should get easily removed by rinsing.
2. It should be capable of removing soil, excessive sebum and residues of setting lotions, etc.
3. It should provide a pleasant fragrance to the hair.
4. After shampooing it should leave the hair in soft and lustrous condition.
5. Shampoo should impart a sufficient degree of foam to satisfy the 'user'.
6. It should be non-toxic and non-irritant.

Shampoos are of different types like, clear lotions, pastes, gels, aerosols, dry products, etc.

Raw materials which are used for the preparation of shampoos are detergents/surfactants and other additives. Detergents are added to impart foaming and cleansing action. They can be of different types, e.g., anionic, cationic and non-ionic detergents. These materials form the base of shampoos. Additives include foam builders, conditioning agents, opacifying agents, clarifying agents, antidandruff agents, preservatives, perfumes, etc. Foam builders are added to the formulation to increase quality, volume and stability of lather, e.g., dodecyl benzene sulfonate, lauroyl monoethanolamide, etc. Conditioning agent helps in lubricating hair and improves handling properties of hair fibre, e.g., lanolin and its derivatives, glycerol and propylene glycol. Sulphur, salicylic acid, hexachlorophene act as antidandruff agents. To preserve the shampoos against bacteria or mould contamination, preservatives like butylated hydroxy benzoate, phenylmercuric nitrate, formaldehyde, etc., are added.

Formulae :

1. Liquid shampoo

Coconut oil	14	%
Olive oil	3	%
Castor oil	3	%
Potassium hydroxide	5.3	%
Glycerol	2	%
Ethyl alcohol	4	%
Sodium hexametaphosphate	1	%
Perfume	0.3	%
Water	68	%

2. Cream shampoo

Calcium alginate	2	%
Sodium citrate	1	%
Triethanolamine lauryl sulphate	10	%
Glycerol	5	%
Methyl paraben	0.15	%
Perfume	0.85	%
Water	81	%

Shampoos can be evaluated by their performance properties and product characteristics.

Hair Dressings

Hair dressings or creams or brilliantines are applied to dry hair in order to provide extra gloss/sheen. Their main purpose is to apply a thin film of oil to keep the hair in order and to give a natural-looking gloss without any appearance of oiliness. Hair dressings can be categorised according to their usage, whether they are intended for men or women.

Women's hair dressings

1. Mucilage lotions
2. Resin lotions
3. Heated curlers
4. Hair sprays

Men's hair dressings

1. Brilliantines (liquid and solid)
2. Non-oily fixatives
3. Emulsions (o/w and w/o types)
4. Gels
5. Aerosols

Hair setting lotions or mucilage lotions are used by women to keep the hair style in a set position in which it has been placed. These lotions are based on gums (tragacanth or acacia) and mucilage. Alcohol is added to decrease the drying time and for wetting purposes. Nowadays resin lotions are more commonly used. They contain polyvinylpyrrolidone, polyethylene glycol and alcohol, etc.

Generally hair dressings consist of combination of oil and water in various forms. Brilliantines are used by men to keep their hair in order and to improve its lustre. Cream brilliantines contain waxes, mineral oils, and stearic acid, etc. Waxes impart extra gloss to the hair while mineral oil helps in maintaining viscosity of cream. As w/o creams get separated on storage, suitable emulsifying agents like fatty acid soaps, wool alcohols, calcium hydroxide with fatty acid, etc., are added.

Emulsions are very popular particularly in western countries because of their more fixative property. Gels are of two types :

1. Microgels
2. True gels

Microgels are transparent o/w emulsions while true gels are aqueous polyethylene glycol solution.

Aerosol hair dressings should have pourable viscosity. It should not be brittle. It should be easily combed and shampooed out.

Formulae :

Hair dressing lotion

1. Gum tragacanth   1.2 %
   Alcohol   10   %
   Glycerin   5   %
   Water   83.8 %
   Preservative q.s.

2. Mineral oil   66%
   Peanut oil   34%
   Colour perfume q.s.

3. Polyethylene glycol   20%
   Water   20%
   Alcohol   59%
   Resin (PVP)   1%
   Colour perfume q.s.

4. Mineral oil   45%
   Oleic acid   12%
   Bees wax   2%
   Lanolin   2%
   Lime water   19%
   Saccharated lime water   20%
   Perfume and preservative q.s.

Hair Removers

Unwanted hair can be removed by two methods :

1. Epilation
2. Depilation

Epilation involves uprooting of intact hair which is very painful and may cause serious skin damage. It can be done by plucking, electrolysis, etc. But nowadays certain epilatory preparations are used in modified form containing mineral oil, wax, rosin, etc.

The term depilation is used nowadays for removal of superfluous hair without causing an injury or pain. For this chemical substances like inorganic sulphides and thioglycollates, etc., are used. An ideal depilatory should possess following properties :

1. It should be non-toxic and non-irritant to the skin.
2. It should be capable of removing hair in 4-6 minutes.

3. It should be economical, stable and easy to apply.
4. It should be odourless and perfumed.
5. It should not leave any stains.

Depilatory preparations usually contain alkaline reducing agents which make the hair fibres swell and ultimately help in cleavage of cystine bridges for complete removal of hair. The chemicals used in the preparation of depilatory are sulphides, stannites, substituted mercaptans, thioglycollates, etc. In addition to this a depilatory preparation contains humectants (glycerin or sorbitol), thickening agent (methyl cellulose) and perfume, etc.

Sulphides are less popular because of production of strong odour of hydrogen sulphide on application. Although 2% aqueous solution of sodium sulphide will disintegrate hair within 6-7 minutes but simultaneously it will damage stratum corneum.

Stannites have no appreciable odour but they form stannates (instability with water, hence stabilizers are added along with them).

Number of depilatories today contain substituted mercaptans which are used along with alkaline reacting materials. They have safer action without producing bad odour, e.g., calcium thioglycollate with calcium hydroxide.

Thioglycollate based preparations are more stable and non-toxic at a concentration between 2.5-4%. They provide depilation effect at a pH not less than 10 and time of depilation varies from 5-15 minutes according to pH. They are generally used in paste form containing chalk, thickening agent, etc.

Depilatories are available in powder, lotion, cream and paste forms. They are packed in jars, collapsible tubes made of plastic and other suitable non-reactive materials.

Formula :

Calcium thioglycollate	7	%
Calcium hydroxide	7	%
Calcium carbonate precipitated	20	%
Cetyl alcohol	5	%
Sodium lauryl sulphate	1	%
Sodium silicate solution	2.5	%
Water perfume q.s.		

10

Sterile Dosage Forms

Definition

Parenteral preparations (injectables) are the sterile solutions or suspensions of drugs in aqueous or oily vehicles meant for introduction into the body by means of an injectable needle under or through one or more layers of skin or mucous membrane. Injectables should be sterile, isotonic and should be free from particles like dust, fibres. Parenteral preparations are used for a number of purposes. They may be used for rapid onset of action, e.g., emergency administration of morphine or penicillin. They must be introduced through the same route for which they are intended, e.g., oily suspensions should always be given by intra-muscular route.

Advantages

1. For immediate physiological action of the drug in emergency, intra-venous route of administration is followed.
2. Modified form of the drug can be given by this route to slow and prolong the action of the drug.
3. Drug can be administered parenterally when they cannot be given orally in case of unconscious and uncooperative state of patient.
4. Amount of solution to be administered can be varied from millilitres to litres.
5. This route has advantage when the drugs get inactivated in G.I.T. or drugs are not well absorbed after oral administration.

Disadvantages

1. Trained personnel are always required to administer the drugs.
2. Injection causes pain at the site of injection.
3. Aseptic conditions and proper sterilisation is necessary for parenteral products.
4. The administration of a drug through wrong route of injection may prove fatal.
5. It becomes difficult to save a patient when overdose is given.

General requirements for parenteral dosage form

Ideal requirements for parenteral products are as follows :

1. They should be free from living microbes.
2. Freedom from microbial products such as toxins, pyrogens.
3. They should be isotonic, i.e., their osmotic pressure should be the same as that of body fluids.
4. They should be free from physical and chemical contaminants.
5. Their specific gravity should match that of body fluids.

Types of Parenteral Formulations

On the basis of physical characters, the injectables can be classified as follows :

1. Injectables in solution form.
2. Injectables in emulsion form.
3. Injectables in suspension form.
4. Dry soluble products which are dissolved in a suitable solvent immediately before its administration.
5. Dry insoluble products which are combined with a suitable vehicle before its administration.

On the basis of route of administration, the parenterals can be classified as under :

1. Intracutaneous or intradermal injections.
2. Subcutaneous or hypodermic injections.
3. Intramuscular injections.
4. Intravenous injections.
5. Intra-arterial injections.
6. Intracardiac injections.
7. Intrathecal injections.
8. Intracisternal injections.
9. Intracerebral injections.
10. Intra-articular injections.

Formulation of Parenterals

Formulation of parenterals require clear understanding of principles regarding accuracy, measurements, cleanliness and quality control of the product. It should be kept in mind that such dosage forms should include minimum number of additives in smallest possible quantities. These substances are :

1. Vehicles
2. Adjuvants
    (a) Solubilising agents
    (b) Stabilizers
    (c) Buffers
    (d) Tonicity factors
    (e) Wetting, suspending and emulsifying agents
    (f) Antimicrobial agents
    (g) Chelating agents

1. Vehicles

Aqueous and non-aqueous vehicles are used for injectables.

Aqueous vehicle

Water is used as a vehicle for number of preparations because it is well tolerated by the body and safest to administer. The aqueous vehicles used are :

 (i) water for injection
 (ii) water for injection free from CO_2
 (iii) water for injection free from dissolved air.

Water for injection

It is a sterile water free from pyrogens, volatile and non-volatile impurities. Pyrogens are thermostable, non-volatile by-products of micro-organisms. Chemically they are polysaccharides and can pass through bacteria-proof filters. For making it free from pyrogens, simple distillation in which an efficient trap is used to prevent the entry of pyrogens into the condenser, is done. Water for injection containing pyrogens causes rise in body temperature, hence test for pyrogens is performed to ensure it to be pyrogen free.

Non-aqueous vehicle

Commonly used non-aqueous vehicles are oils and alcohols. Oily vehicles are generally used when

1. a delayed absorption of medicament is required;
2. the medicament is not stable in water;
3. the drug is soluble in oil.

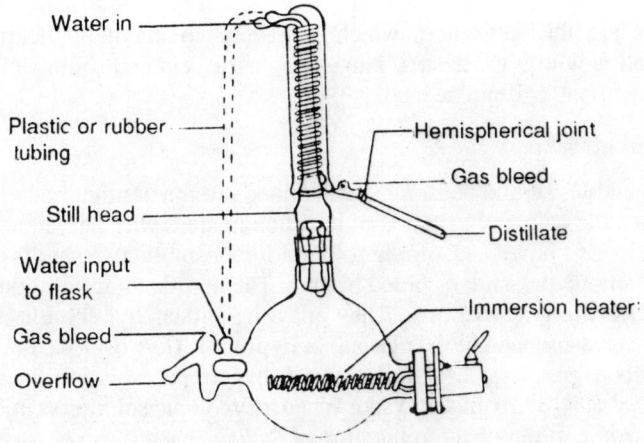

Water in

Plastic or rubber tubing

Still head

Water input to flask

Gas bleed

Overflow

Hemispherical joint

Gas bleed

Distillate

Immersion heater

Fig. 10.1. Water still.

Examples : arachis oil, cotton seed oil, almond oil, sesame oil. In addition to this, other non-aqueous vehicles are ethyl alcohol, glycerin, propylene glycol, etc.

2. Adjuvants

Adjuvants are added to improve the quality and stability of parenterals. These agents should be physically and chemically compatible with the entire formulation. They should be non-toxic and should be added in minimum possible quantity.

(a) Solubilising agents

These agents are added to increase the solubility of poorly soluble/ insoluble drugs. The solubility of such medicaments can be increased by complex formation and by using cosolvents, surfactants (tweens, spans).

(b) Stabilizers

These substances are added in the formulation to prevent oxidation and hydrolysis of the medicament. To prevent oxidation either a suitable antioxidant is used or the product is sealed in a container from which oxygen has already been replaced. The examples of suitable antioxidants are sodium metabisulphite, ascorbic acid, thiourea, tocopherol, sodium bisulphite. Hydrolysis can be prevented either by replacing a part or whole of water in the preparation by a non-aqueous solvent.

(c) Buffers

Buffers are the substances which are added to maintain the pH of preparation within the desired range, e.g., citric acid and sodium citrate, acetic acid and sodium acetate.

(d) Tonicity factors

All injectables should be isotonic with blood plasma or other body fluids to reduce the pain and irritation of injection in areas with nerve endings. A solution is known as **isotonic** solution if its osmotic pressure is equal to the osmotic pressure of blood plasma. The non-isotonic solutions are called **paratonic** solutions. They may be either **hypertonic** (high osmotic pressure than blood plasma) or **hypotonic** (low osmotic pressure than blood plasma). I.V. injection of hypertonic solution leads to shrinkage of R.B.C. (plasmolysis). When a hypotonic solution is injected by I.V. route, it may lead to bursting of R.B.C. (haemolysis).

The isotonicity of a solution is adjusted by using dextrose, sodium chloride and sodium sulphate, etc.

(e) Wetting, suspending and emulsifying agents

Table 10.1.

S. No.	Name	Purpose of addition	Examples
1.	Wetting agent	To reduce the interfacial energy between the solid particle and the liquid.	Tween 80, sorbitan trioleate
2.	Suspending agent	To improve the viscosity and to suspend the particles for a long time.	Methyl cellulose, carboxy methyl cellulose, gelatin
3.	Emulsifying agent	They are generally used in sterile emulsions.	Lecithin

(f) Antimicrobial agents

These substances in bacteriostatic or fungistatic concentration must be added in multidose containers. These substances prevent the growth of micro-organisms and act as preservatives. Antimicrobial agents must be studied well with respect to compatibility with other components of the preparation. Among the commonly used antibacterial agents are :

1. Phenol (0.5% w/v)
2. Cresol (0.3% w/v)
3. Chlorocresol (0.1% w/v)

4. Phenylmercuric acetate (0.001% w/v)
5. Phenylmercuric nitrate (0.001% w/v)
6. Benzalkonium chloride (0.01%)

(g) *Chelating agents*

Chelating agents are added to chelate the metallic ion and form a complex which gets dissolved in the solvent, e.g., EDTA (ethylene diamine tetra-acetic acid) and its salts, sodium or potassium salts of citric acid, etc.

Processing of Parenteral Products

In the preparation of parenteral products, there are numerous requirements which should be taken into consideration. Environment requires careful monitoring and control in which the various stages of production take place. There are three main sources of contamination which should be controlled to make the surrounding environment free from microbial contamination and comparatively particulate free. These contaminants are :

(i) Atmosphere

(ii) Apparatus and handling devices

(iii) Personnel

(i) *Atmosphere*

The air in this area must be free from dust particles and micro-organism. Air from outside is passed through HEPA filters (high efficiency particulate air) which can remove particles up to 0.3 μ. For the control of personnel, air conditioning and humidity control should be incorporated to the system. HEPA filters make use of laminar air flow in which air moves with uniform velocity of about 30 metres/min. In the laminar flow system, the air flows in parallel with minimum turbulence. The entire area should be constructed in such a manner that it can be easily cleaned and disinfected. Furniture should be minimum for ease in disinfection. Suitable air lock system should be provided by which objects and personnel can pass into and out of the work area. Stainless steel is the best material which allows adequate and regular cleaning of surfaces and is resistant to chemicals used for disinfection. Ultraviolet rays have an antibacterial action, thereby producing a disinfectant action. But direct exposure to personnel may cause irritation to skin and particularly eyes of human beings, therefore they must be protected.

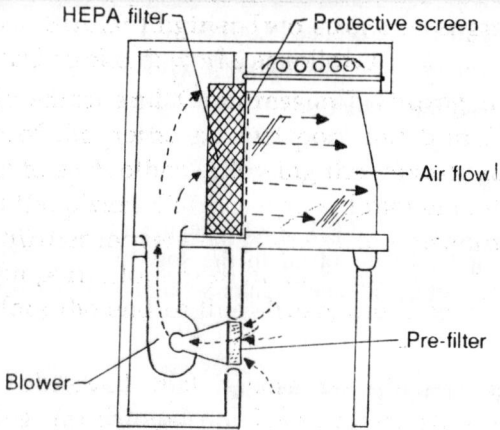

Fig. 10.2. Horizontal laminar air flow workbench.

(ii) *Apparatus and handling devices*

As far as apparatus is concerned, each apparatus which is likely to come in contact with products must be sterile. This requirement is very essential when preparation is to be handled under aseptic conditions because the entry of a single micro-organism will spoil the whole product. Clarification is achieved by passing the solutions under different pressures through filters like sintered glass filter and membrane filters. The final containers have also to be pre-sterilised and the products have to be transferred under aseptic conditions.

(iii) *Personnel*

The quality of parenteral products is critically dependent upon personnel employed. Considerable stress should be given on personal hygiene of the worker because they could prove to be the greatest source of particulate and microbial contamination. Hence they should always wear special sterile clothing, including hoods and gloves. The garment should be of textiles that shed minimum fibres. Air showers are sometimes directed on personnel before entering aseptic area. Their footwear should also be covered with sterilisable and disposable covers.

Preparation of Parenteral Products

The following steps are involved in the preparation of parenteral products :

1. Cleaning of equipment, containers and closures.
2. Preparation of solution/suspension.
3. Filtration.

4. Fillings of the product in ampoules/vials.
5. Sealing.
6. Sterilisation.
7. Tests for quality control.
8. Labelling and packing.

1. *Cleaning of equipment, containers and closures*

Equipments and containers used for parenteral preparations are cleaned with detergent solution and washed with tap water first, followed by distilled water and water for injection. Rubber closures are washed with hot solution of 0.5% sodium pyrophosphate in water. After washing they are sterilised in an autoclave or hot air oven.

2. *Preparation of solution/suspension*

The product to be prepared may be in the form of an aqueous solution or oily solution or suspension. Therefore various ingredients of formulation are collected at one place where compounding is to be done. It should be kept in mind that solution must be prepared under aseptic conditions.

3. *Filtration*

If the solution contains any foreign particle, it must be filtered through bacteria-proof filters such as seitz filters, membrane filters and sintered glass filters.

4. *Filling of the product in ampoules/vials*

The filtered product is filled into ampoules/vials with the help of semi-automatic or automatic machines under aseptic conditions. On small scale filling can be done with hypodermic syringes attached with long needles, burettes, etc. While filling ampoules precaution should be taken that the needle does not touch the neck of the ampoule to prevent cracking and staining at the time of sealing.

5. *Sealing*

Sealing should be done immediately after filling under aseptic conditions only. Sealing of ampoules can be done by fusion of glass in hot flame of blast or torch but nowadays automatic machines are available for large scale production. Vials and bottles are sealed by fitting the rubber closure with the help of vacuum and then aluminium cap is further placed on it either by hand or by mechanical method.

6. Sterilisation

Sterilisation is done by various methods depending upon nature of preparation. In case of thermostable drugs, sterilisation is carried out either in autoclave at a temperature of 115-116°C for 30 minutes or in an oven at 150-160°C for one hour. For thermolabile drugs, sterilisation is done by filtration through bacteria-proof filters. In case of oily vehicle, the sterilisation is done by dry heat method.

7. Tests for quality control

Following tests are performed to maintain quality of parenterals :

    (i) Sterility test

   (ii) Clarity test

  (iii) Leakage test

  (iv) Pyrogen test

   (v) Assay

8. Labelling

The label should be complete with all necessary informations like

    (i) Name of product

   (ii) Volume of product

  (iii) Route of administration

  (iv) Batch No., Mfg. lic. No.

   (v) Date of manufacture

  (vi) Date of expiry

 (vii) Storage

(viii) Dose, use

  (ix) Manufacturer's address

   (x) Retail price

Total Parenteral Nutrition (TPN)

It involves the fulfillment of patient's nutritional requirements by the intravenous route. TPN is given to increase the chance of patient's survival in pre-operative and post-operative conditions. Generally, TPN solution consists of mixture of amino acids, lipid emulsion, electrolytes and vitamins with trace elements.

Amino acids are the most accessible source of nitrogen and are required for protein formation because the whole proteins are not accepted by those patients. TPN solution also provides calories from a non-nitrogenous source, e.g., dextrose, sorbitol. Lipid emulsion of essential fatty acid (e.g., linoleic acid) is generally given at intervals of

2 or 3 days to satisfy the requirements. Water soluble vitamins (e.g., vitamin B) are also present in TPN solution.

TPN products are generally administered to avoid multiple injections. Administration through a peripheral vein is ideal for TPN because it requires relatively uncomplicated procedure.

Sometimes they may be hypertonic and may cause irritation to the tissues.

I.V. Admixtures

Nowadays there is widespread practice of mixing drugs to infusion fluids. These additions are often performed by nurses by injecting the drug through rubber closure. This may lead to the following :

(i) *Microbial contamination*

As there is no bactericide in I.V. infusions and they contain sugar and amino acid which may support bacterial growth after addition of the drug therefore addition should always be done aseptically.

(ii) *Incompatibility*

Physical, chemical and therapeutical incompatibilities may occur due to the interaction between additives and infusion. Physical incompatibility will show change in colour, crystallization, precipitation, etc., while chemical incompatibility cannot be detected visually and is often due to change in pH, e.g., if the pH of dextrose solution containing ampicillin is greater than 5.0, the combination is incompatible. Similarly, potassium penicillin G contains a citrate buffer and is buffered at pH 6.0 to 6.5 to ensure the activity of the antibiotic even if it is intravenously admixtured with dextrose or sodium chloride injection.

Following are the few methods for safe and effective use of I.V. admixture in hospitals :

1. Proper training should be given to nurses and pharmacists for preparation of admixtures.
2. Nurses should be instructed that whenever a drug is added to an infusion fluid, a label must be attached bearing "Date and time of addition and quantity of added drug".
3. Hospital pharmacy department should provide latest informations regarding drug stability and compatibility to the paramedical staff.
4. As far as possible the hospital pharmacist should avoid addition of medicaments to infusion bottles by adopting other suitable formulations.

Dialysis Fluids

In renal failure, it becomes essential to remove the waste products and to maintain electrolyte balance. This can be done either by haemodialysis or intraperitoneal dialysis method.

1. Haemodialysis

Composition of haemodialysis solution :

   (a)   Dextrose monohydrate — to give 0.1-0.2% strength after dilution
   (b)   Sodium acetate
   (c)   Lactic acid
   (d)   Various ionic substances like sodium, potassium, calcium, magnesium bicarbonates and/or chlorides.

Method of preparation

First dissolve calcium, magnesium salts, potassium chloride and lactic acid in about 70% of the final volume of water. To this add sodium chloride, sodium acetate and dextrose. The solution is then filtered and packed in large plastic containers.

Method

Haemodialysis is done by using an artificial kidney. In this, the blood from an artery is led into a machine in which it is separated from the dialysis fluid by a semi-permeable membrane. This membrane is permeable to urea, electrolytes and dextrose but not to plasma proteins and lipids. Certain substances which are present in excess quantity in the blood pass out into the fluid while the deficiencies are made up in the blood by this method only. After treatment, the blood is freed from air bubbles and clots and pumped back into the patient via suitable vein. A kidney unit may require more than 1200 litres of solution a week. Concentrated solutions can be diluted with deionised water, or distilled water, soft water.

2. Intraperitoneal dialysis

Composition of intraperitoneal dialysis solution

Intraperitoneal dialysis solution must be sterile so that the pyrogens may not penetrate peritoneal membrane. They have got similar composition to haemodialysis solution except in the following respects :

   (i)   There is no potassium ion. If required, potassium chloride can be added separately.
   (ii)   Anhydrous dextrose is used instead of dextrose monohydrate.

(iii) As they are ready for use, they are much more dilute and always contain magnesium and calcium ions.

(iv) Solvent used is water for injection.

(v) Two grades of dextrose are used. One is approx. 1.4% and the other 7% for rapid reduction of oedema.

Commercial solutions sometimes contain lactate also. As these solutions are dilute solutions, no special method of preparation is required.

Method

This requires irrigation of peritoneal cavity with dialysis solution and in this peritoneum acts as a semi-permeable membrane. Conventional method allows the entry of the contents (already warmed) of bottles into the peritoneal cavity via a common catheter passed through the abdominal wall. It requires approximately 10 minutes and after half an hour, the bottles are lowered to allow the liquid to drain out. After some time again the cycle is repeated with fresh fluid. A complete intra-peritoneal dialysis requires about 25 cycles (i.e., 50 bottles) in about 36 hours.

Quality Control of Parenterals

1. Sterility testing

All the parenteral preparations must comply with the official test for sterility I.P. That means the product should be free from living micro-organisms and their spores.

Principle

Sample to be tested is transferred into test tube containing sterile culture media under aseptic condition for the growth of aerobic and anaerobic micro-organism. The growth can be detected easily because the clear medium turns turbid. Following culture media are used :

1. Fluid thioglycollate medium (for detection of aerobic and anaerobic bacteria);

2. Soyabean casein digest medium (for detection of fungi and aerobic bacteria).

Controls

The following controls should also be done along with the test for sterility :

1. *First control*

The medium for the detection of bacteria is incubated at 30-35°C for 7 days. Similarly the medium for detection of fungi is incubated at 20-25°C for 7 days. If the media is sterile, there should be no growth.

2. *Second control*

Each medium is incubated at the required temperature for 7 days after adding a suspension of micro-organism to it. Suspension of aerobe, anaerobe and fungi are added separately to each of the media. Early and copious growth of micro-organisms proves that the media is capable of supporting microbial growth at prevailing conditions.

3. *Third control*

Here each medium is incubated in two portions. To both the portions is added a suspension of an aerobe, or a suspension of an anaerobe or a suspension of a fungus respectively. To one portion is added a quantity of the parenteral preparation under test. After incubation for not more than 7 days at 35°C there should be early and copious growth proving that the parenteral preparation does not have any antimicrobial activity.

Test for sterility

The test can be performed by using either method A or method B in a sterile atmosphere.

Method A (membrane filtration method)

In this sterile membrane filter of pore size 0.45 μ is used in a sterilised filter unit. Sterile fluid A (dil. solution of peptic digest in water) is added in sufficient quantity to moisten the membrane.

If the parenteral preparation to be tested is an aqueous solution, the prescribed quantity is drawn through the filter. If the solution being tested is antimicrobial, wash the membrane by running through it 3 successive quantities of 100 ml each of fluid A so that the antimicrobial ingredient is either completely washed out or reduced to a very low non-inhibitory concentration. Either two membranes can be used, one for each test or one membrane can be used. In the latter case the membrane is divided into two equal halves, one for each test.

One membrane or one half of the membrane is removed aseptically and put into 100 ml of fluid thioglydrate medium and incubated at 30-35°C for not less than seven days. The other membrane or the other half of the membrane is immersed in 100 ml of soyabean casein digest medium and incubated at 20-25°C for not less than 7 days.

Oils, oily solutions and ointments may be diluted or dissolved in a suitable sterile diluent such as isopropyl myristate (not an antimicrobial) and filtered through the membrane filter. The membrane is washed by filtering through it three successive quantities of 100 ml each of sterile fluid B (which is only fluid A to which polysorbate 80 has been added). Polysorbate 80 ensures solution of the oily or greasy substance in fluid A. Afterwards the same procedure is followed as stated for aqueous solution.

Method B (direct inoculation method)

For aqueous solutions and suspensions the prescribed quantity of liquid is drawn through a sterile pipette or with a sterile syringe and needle. It is transferred and mixed with the medium under aseptic conditions. The media is then incubated at the specified temperature for not less than 14 days.

If the material being tested makes the medium turbid, suitable portion of the medium is transformed to fresh medium between the third and seventh day of incubation. Both old and fresh medias are incubated for a total of 14 days.

In case of oils and oily suspensions being tested, a sterile emulsifying agent without antimicrobial activity such as polysorbate 80 is added to the medium to help in the emulsification and easy mixing of oil in the medium.

Ointments are diluted with sterile fluid B and the solution is mixed with the medium. In both the cases, the medias are incubated for not less than 14 days.

Interpretation of results

If no growth is found during the incubation period or at the end of it, the preparation being tested passes the test.

If growth is found and if it can be shown that it is due to some contaminant during the course of the sterility testing and not because the preparation is not sterile, the test may be repeated in the same way. If no growth is found, the material or preparation passes the test.

If growth is found, a second re-test is allowed under certain conditions. If again growth appears, the preparation fails the test.

2. Pyrogen test

This test is performed to check the presence or absence of pyrogens in all aqueous parenteral products. Rabbits are used to perform this test because their body temperature increases when pyrogens (external stimuli) are introduced in their bodies by parenteral route.

For this test, three healthy rabbits are selected each weighing at least 1.5 kg. No rabbit is selected if

(i) it has a normal temperature greater than 49.8°C;

(ii) it was used in a positive test during the last two weeks or in a negative test during the last 2 days.

If the animals are used for the first time, to get accustomed to this test, 'sham test' is carried out. For this I.V. injection of 10 ml/kg body wt. normal saline is injected into them. Any animal showing a rise in temperature of 0.6°C or more is rejected for the test.

Test for pyrogen

The test is carried out in an air-conditioned room. During the test food is withheld to the rabbits overnight and water is withheld. Clinical thermometer is inserted as temperature recording device into the rectum of each rabbit to a depth of not less than 7.5 cm. Two normal readings of rectal temperature should be taken prior to the test injection at an interval of half an hour and the mean of these two is calculated. This is called initial temperature.

Needles, glassware, syringes, etc., to be used for this test should be made pyrogen-free by first washing with water for injection and heating in an air oven at 250°C for one hour. The test injection is warmed to 38°C and injected slowly through an ear vein in a dose of 0.5 to 10 ml per kg of rabbit weight. Rectal temperature readings are then recorded at an interval of half an hour till six readings.

Interpretation of results

The response of each rabbit can be detected by subtracting the initial temperature from the maximum temperature, which is the highest temperature recorded. Addition of three responses from three rabbits gives the sum of the responses. If the sum dose not exceed 1.4°C and if the response of any individual rabbit is less than 0.6°C, the preparation passes the test. If the sum is more than 1.4°C or if the response of any individual rabbit is 0.6°C or more, continue the test using 5 other rabbits. Again if sum of all rabbits is less than 3.7°C and if the individual response of not more than three rabbits is 0.6°C or more, the preparation being tested passes the test.

3. Particulate matter monitoring

Particulate matter in parenteral products is defined as unwanted mobile insoluble matter. The particles larger than the size of R.B.C. are very dangerous because they may block the blood vessels which may lead to serious results.

Particulate matter may enter from number of sources which can be classified as :

(i) intrinsic contamination — materials originally present in the solution;

(ii) extrinsic contamination — materials from the environment (shedding from the body and clothes of the person, ceilings, walls and furniture of room).

Methods for monitoring particulate matter contamination

(i) Visual method

This test is performed by holding the neck of filled container against strongly illuminated screen. Then it is slowly rotated, inverted and examined to exclude the possibility of foreign particles. If any particulate matter is visible, that injection is rejected. Inspectors should not perform inspection for more than two hours at a time.

(ii) Filtration

This method is meant for counting particles in hydraulic fluids. It involves passing the liquid samples through a filter and examine the material collected on the surface of filter under a microscope. This method requires skilled and highly trained technicians. The only difficulty in this method is with oily particles because oil tends to become absorbed into the membrane filter and particles are not measured.

(iii) Light blockage

This method gives an automatic evaluation of particulate in hydraulic oils. It allows a stream of the fluid to be tested to pass between a bright white light source and a photodiode sensor. This instrument is able to detect the cross-sectional area of the particle because it blocks out the path of light and size of particle is considered as a diameter of a circle of equivalent area.

(iv) Coulter counter

Coulter counter is based on the principle that increase in resistance is observed between two electrodes (either side of an orifice) as the particle approaches and passes through the orifice. It requires addition of an electrolyte prior to evaluation. It can detect particles with diameter below 0.1 μm.

4. Faulty seals packaging

Validity of closure integrity is of vital importance to parenteral preparation. Therefore, following tests can be performed :

(i) *Leakage test*

This test is performed only for ampoules which have been sealed by fusion method to see that the ampoules are sealed properly and they may not leak to the outside to spoil the package. If sealing is not perfect the contents may get deteriorated by atmospheric contaminants.

Leakage test is performed in a vacuum chamber (by producing a negative pressure). Ampoules are dipped in 1% sodium methylene blue solution in vacuum chamber and vacuum is applied. After some time vacuum is released and the entry of dye to the parenteral preparation is checked. The presence of dye in the ampoule confirms the leakage and hence rejected. Generally autoclaving of ampoules is done in a dye bath. Vials and bottles are not subjected to this test because the sealing material used is not rigid.

(ii) *Spark detector method*

When the product is thermolabile (e.g., vaccines), leakage can be tested using a spark detector. A spark across a high voltage source is observed whenever there is any leakage in the container or sometimes if the ampoules are filled with an inert gas the glow inside the ampoule will indicate integrity.

11

Ophthalmic Products

Ophthalmic products are the sterile products either meant for instillation into the space between the eyelids and the eye balls or for topical application. Ophthalmic products can be classified as under :

(a) Eye drops

(b) Eye ointments

(c) Eye lotions

(d) Eye packs

(e) Eye discs

(f) Contact lens solution

Essential characteristics of different ophthalmic preparations

Ophthalmic preparations should possess the following properties :

1. *Sterility*

Ophthalmic preparation must be sterile when prepared. A gram negative bacillus *Pseudomonas aeruginosa* is found to be present frequently in ophthalmic products which may cause serious infection of cornea. It can cause complete loss of sight in 24-28 hours. This organism is a common inhabitant of skin which may come from the physician, the patient, the nurse or from the air. The other organisms which are also responsible for infection of ophthalmic tissues are *Bacillus subtilis*, *Aspergillus fungigatus* and viruses.

Ophthalmic products when packed in multidose containers get contaminated if the tip of dropper touches the surface of eyelid or eyelash during instillation. Hence it becomes essential to add antimicrobial compounds to preserve ophthalmic preparations. The preservative should be non-toxic, non-irritant, and should be compatible with medicament. Ophthalmic preparations can be sterilised using following methods :

(i) By autoclaving

(ii) By filtration method

(iii) Addition of antimicrobial substances at lower temperatures.

Chapter 11

2. Tonicity

Ophthalmic products must be isotonic with lachrymal secretions to avoid discomfort and irritation. However, it has been found that eyes can tolerate a range of tonicity from 0.5% to 2% sodium chloride before discomfort is experienced. There are some isotonic vehicles which are used to prepare ophthalmic products like 1.9% w/v boric acid which is isotonic with lachrymal secretion and has a pH slightly below 5.0. It is found to be suitable for salts of procaine, phenylephrine and zinc. U.S.P. recommends inclusion of phenylmercuric nitrate in boric acid vehicles as a preservative. Similarly a group of 10 solutions, known as Sorensen phosphate buffer, has pH range 5.9-8.0. It has been stated in pharmacopoeia that solution having a pH of 6.8 is the best suitable for ephedrine, atropine, pilocarpine, etc.

Now drugs are added to the above mentioned vehicles which make them hypertonic. If the quantity of drug added is small, the net effect is slight/negligible but if the quantity is in appreciable amounts, we have to modify the method of preparation.

3. pH of the preparation

pH plays a very important role in therapeutic activity, solubility, stability and comfort to the patient. Tears have a pH of about 7.4. Eyes can tolerate solution having wide range of pH values from 3.5-10 provided they are not strongly buffered since the tears will rapidly restore the normal pH value of the eye, e.g., alkaloidal salt solutions are stable at pH 2-3 but this pH is irritant to the eyes and moreover alkaloids get precipitated at pH above 7 which gives rise to problems. Hence pH of ophthalmic preparation must be monitored carefully.

4. Surface activity

Vehicles used in ophthalmic preparation must have wetting ability to penetrate cornea and other tissues. Therefore certain surfactants or wetting agents are added which are found suitable for ophthalmic products and they will not cause any damage to tissues of eye. Examples : Benzalkonium chloride, polysorbate 20, polysorbate 80, dioctylsodium sulfosuccinate, etc.

5. Viscosity

To prolong the contact time of the drug in the eye various thickening agents are added. These agents improve viscosity of preparation and thus therapeutic effect. They should have following properties :

1. Easy to be filtered.
2. Easy to be sterilised.

3. They must have requisite refractive index and clarity.

4. They should be compatible with other ingredients.

Examples : cellulose derivatives (methyl cellulose, carboxymethyl cellulose, hydroxy propyl methyl cellulose, hydroxy propyl ethyl cellulose), synthetic polymers (polyvinyl alcohol, polyethylene glycols).

Thickening agents are not added in drops or lotions which are meant for use during or after surgery due to some possible adverse effects on the interior of the eye.

6. *Clarity*

All ophthalmic products must be clear and free from foreign particles, fibres and filaments.

This absolute clarity can be obtained by suitable filtration methods. The best filtration medium is microporous plastic membrane (0.8 μm pore size). The use of sintered glass disc mounted on a buchner funnel has the advantage that it neither absorbs any solution nor furnishes any fibres or particles to the filtrate. Filter paper and absorbent cotton are rarely used. If at all a filter paper is to be used, it must be hard surfaced Whatman filter paper No. 54. For cotton, highest grade cotton should be selected. Medicaments in suspension should be in an ultra-fine state of subdivision to minimise irritation. If different ophthalmic products are to be prepared, separate filter for each solution should be used to avoid the possibility of contamination.

Eye Drops

Eye drops are sterile aqueous or oily solutions or suspensions meant for instillation into the conjunctival sac. They require additives like :

1. Vehicles (aqueous or oily vehicles)

Oily vehicles are rarely used to dissolve hydrophobic drugs, e.g., peanut oil is used to dissolve di-isopropyl fluorophosphate.

2. Buffers

Buffers are added for adjustment of pH so as to reduce discomfort, to maintain chemical stability and to improve clinical response. Examples : boric acid solution, isotonic phosphate buffer.

3. Tonicity adjusting substances

Eye drops are made isotonic with lachrymal secretion with the help of various buffers and other solutions.

4. Viscosity builders

Thickening agent like hypomellose is commonly used which gives clear solution and sheds few fibres.

5. Preservatives

Generally eye drops are prepared in aqueous vehicles, therefore bactericides or fungicides must be added to preserve eye drops. Preservatives used are phenyl mercuric nitrate or acetate (0.002%), benzalkonium chlorides (0.01%), chlorhexidine acetate (0.01%), chlorocresol (0.05%), chlorbutol (0.5%), thiomersal (0.01%).

6. Anti-oxidants

They are added in several eye drops to give protection against atmospheric oxygen. This protection can be further improved by replacing the air in the container with an inert gas. Examples : sodium metabisulphite, sodium thiosulphate.

7. Wetting agents

Various wetting agents are used for proper penetration of eye drops into the cornea. Examples : dioctylsodium sulfosuccinate, polysorbate 80, polysorbate 20, etc.

Special precautions

Special precautions should be taken while handling and storage of eye drops.

Aseptically prepared eye drops must be used within two weeks after first opening of the container because organism may enter during instillation. This is the only reason why eye drops are dispensed in small amounts.

Eye drops should be dispensed in glass or plastic containers attached with suitable dropper for instillation into eye. Care must be taken while handling the eye drops that the nozzle should not touch the 'eye' to avoid contamination. In operation theatres, an unopened new container for each patient is preferred.

Eye drops should be labelled "For external use only." along with storage conditions to maintain full activity, e.g., eye drops containing adrenaline, chloramphenicol must be stored in a cool place. Suspensions must be labelled "Shake the bottle." and "For external use only.". Suspensions must not be allowed to freeze because it may change the crystallinity of the drug which will ultimately affect the bioavailability.

Eye Lotions

Eye lotions or eye washes are sterile isotonic aqueous solutions meant for irrigating the eye cavity to remove foreign particles. They are used with the help of sterile fabric dressing or clean eye bath. Formulation includes various drugs which are used to prepare eye lotions, e.g., sodium chloride, sodium bicarbonate, boric acid, borax or zinc sulphate. Eye lotions are always supplied in concentrated form and are formulated according to the required strength. Lotions are sterilised by autoclaving or filtration.

Special precaution

Containers must be labelled clearly "For external use only." and "Avoid contamination during use and discard any unused part 24 hours after first opening.".

Eye Ointments

Eye ointments are sterile preparations meant for application to the eye. The preparation of ophthalmic ointments must be carried out under aseptic conditions and they are packed in collapsible metal or plastic containers. Nowadays eye applicaps are available which contain one application of the preparation. The common ointment bases used for preparation of eye ointments are yellow soft paraffin, anhydrous lanolin, mineral oil. Emulsion bases containing lanette wax, mineral oil and water are also used. White soft paraffin is not used because it is prepared by bleaching yellow soft paraffin and small proportion of bleaching agent remains there even after careful washing. The container remains sterile provided that it has not been opened.

Contact Lens Solution

They are aqueous solutions meant for lubricating, cleaning and hydrating contact lenses. Contact lenses are made up of polymethyl methacrylate. There are two types of contact lenses.

1. Hard contact lenses
2. Soft contact lenses

1. Hard contact lenses

Hard contact lenses require following two solutions :

(a) Wetting solution

It comprises of wetting agents like polyvinyl alcohol, polysorbate 80, etc., to make the surface of lens hydrophillic and thus ease in insertion.

Buffering agent (boric acid buffers), tonicity adjusters (sodium chloride), thickening agent (cellulose derivatives), and antimicrobials (benzalkonium chloride, chlorhexidine) are also added to prepare wetting solution.

(b) *Storage solutions*

Contact lenses after removal are wetted with wetting solution and rinsed, rubbed well with purified water. Then they are stored in storage solution to prevent dehydration. Storage solution comprises of non-ionic surfactant, and mixture of antimicrobial agents.

2. Soft contact lenses

They are flexible type of lenses. Instructions are given to the persons wearing soft contact lenses to remove them before instilling eye drops. For cleaning soft lenses, they are heated in a 0.9% sodium chloride solution and the solution must be sterile.

Eye Packs

They are used to give prolonged contact of solution with the eye. A cotton pledget is saturated with an ophthalmic solution and this pledget is kept over eye. Packs may provide maximum mydriasis, for example, if saturated with phenylephrine solution.

Eye Discs

These discs generally consist of gel matrices produced in the shape of discs or flakes. Contained drug gets dissolved slowly for a long time after their placement in the eye cavity. Ophthalmic inserts like pilocarpine ocuserts are becoming more popular and it is claimed that they release the drug for 24 hours. They contain a core of pilocarpine and alginic acid. The core is surrounded by ethylene/vinyl acetate copolymer membrane which controls the release of pilocarpine from disc into tear secretion.

12
Tablets

Definition

Tablets are the solid unit dosage forms containing medicament or medicaments with or without suitable diluents. They are prepared either by the process of moulding or by compression method.

Advantages

1. They are easy to handle.
2. They are easy to carry.
3. Bitter taste can be masked by sugar coating or film coating.
4. Measurement of dose is not required.
5. They are easy to swallow.
6. They are more economical.
7. Incompatible drugs can be mixed in tablet dosage form using a buffer layer.
8. They can be chewed or sucked if desired.
9. They are attractive in appearance.
10. They are available in various sizes, shapes and colours, etc.

Formulation of Tablets

Tablets generally consist of number of therapeutically inert substances in addition to medicaments. These substances are known as additives or excipients. They can be classified as follows :

1. Diluents
2. Binding agents
3. Granulating agents
4. Disintegrating agents
5. Lubricants, glidants, anti-adhesive agents
6. Colouring agents
7. Flavouring agents
8. Sweetening agents

1. Diluents

Diluents are added to increase the bulk of the formulation so that the tablet of appropriate size can be prepared. When the quantity of medicament is very small, diluents like lactose, sodium chloride, dextrose, starch, sugar, calcium carbonate, calcium phosphate, etc., are used.

2. Binding agent or binders

These agents are used to impart cohesiveness to powder particles and they give sufficient strength to the granules so as to prevent them from crumbling during transportation. They keep the tablet intact after compression. Various commonly used binding agents are gum acacia, gum tragacanth, starch, gelatin, cellulose, sodium alginate, methyl cellulose, etc. Lozenges and implants require high percentage of binders.

3. Granulating agents

These agents are added to convert fine powder particles into granules. Granulating agents should be present in sufficient concentration. Various commonly used granulating agents are water, alcohol, syrup, mucilages of acacia, tragacanth and starch, etc.

4. Disintegrating agents

They are also known as disintegrants. These substances are added to facilitate the disintegration of tablets in G.I.T. Generally, three types of disintegrating agents are used.

(i) Substances which swell on coming in contact with water, e.g., maize starch, potato starch, sodium alginate, methyl cellulose.

(ii) Substances which produce effervescence when they come in contact with water, e.g., sodium bicarbonate, critic acid, tartaric acid.

(iii) Substances which melt at body temperature, e.g., cocoa butter. A disintegrating agent is generally added in two portions. One part is added to powders before granulation and the other is mixed with granules. The latter portion of disintegrating agent is responsible for breaking the tablet into granules and the first portion helps in breaking the granules into fine particles.

5. Lubricants, glidants, anti-adhesives

Lubricants are added to granules to reduce interparticular friction and to reduce the friction between tablet and die wall, e.g., calcium stearate, magnesium stearate, and talc, etc.

Glidants are added to improve the flow properties of granules from hopper to die, e.g., boric acid, starch, talc, magnesium stearate, etc.

Anti-adhesives are used to prevent adhesion to surfaces of dies and punches (prevent sticking of tablet), e.g., liquid paraffin, stearic acid, calcium stearate, etc.

6. Colouring agents

Colouring agents are added to impart colour, identification and elegance to the tablets. Colour is added in lozenges, chewable tablets, and effervescent tablets, etc. Colouring agent is either mixed with dry powders or may be dissolved in solution used for granulation. The colour should be harmless and approved, e.g., chlorophyll, indigo, flavones, arminic acid, etc.

7. Flavouring agents

These substances are added to impart flavour to lozenges, effervescent tablets, chewable tablets, etc. Flavouring agents are generally volatile in nature, therefore they must be sprayed over the granules before compression, e.g., fruit flavours and volatile oils.

8. Sweetening agents

These substances are added to formulation to improve the taste of tablets and to make them sweet. These agents are used in lozenges and chewable tablets, etc. Some of the common sweetening agents used are mannitol, sucrose and lactose, etc.

PREPARATION OF TABLETS

For preparation of compressed tablet of good quality, fine powders are not used. Either crystalline form or the granules of the ingredients are used for compression. The granules are preferred over fine powders. A comparison of the two is given below :

	Fine powders	Granules
1.	Powders do not flow evenly therefore tablets of varying weights are obtained.	Granules flow evenly through the hopper resulting in the tablets of uniform weight.
2.	Fine powders get separated into layers according to their densities due to vibration of machine.	Granules are uniform in composition and the ingredients are bound together, therefore they cannot separate into layers.

Contd.

Fine powders	*Granules*
3. Chances of air imprisonment is more which may lead to capping of tablet.	Upon compression the granules combine together to form sound tablets.
4. When colour is required in tablets, it is very difficult to mix small amount of colour with so much of the powder.	In case of granules colour can be dissolved in the granulating liquid to distribute the colour uniformly.
5. Fine powder can flow out of the die or hopper easily.	As granules are heavier so they cannot flow out of the die or hopper.

METHODS OF PREPARATION OF TABLETS

There are three methods of preparation of tablets :

1. Direct compression
2. Dry granulation
3. Wet granulation

1. Direct compression method

In this medicament is available in crystalline form which can be passed through required number of sieve and crystals of appropriate size are separated. Then these granules are compressed. But sometimes these tablets do not disintegrate. To overcome this difficulty directly compressible crystalline cellulose and spray dried lactose are added. The drugs which are used for direct compression are potassium chloride, acetylsalicylic acid, etc.

2. Dry granulation method

This is also called slugging, double compression or pre-compression method. It involves dry powder to be compressed into large tablets or slugs with the help of a tablet-making machine. These slugs are then broken into small pieces which are passed through specified sieves. Granules of required size are then mixed with disintegrating agent and lubricant. The granules are then compressed to form tablets.

This method is particularly useful when the medicament is unstable in the presence of moisture.

3. Wet granulation method

This method is most widely used to prepare tablets. The powdered medicament is mixed along with additives like diluent, binding agent, disintegrating agent, etc. The mixture is then moistened with sufficient amount of granulating agent to form a coherent mass. This coherent damp mass is then passed through sieve No. 8 or 10. The wet granules obtained are spread in thin layers in trays and dried at a temperature of 60°C in a hot air oven. The dried granules are passed through sieve No. 20 to get uniformly sized granules. They are then mixed with second portion of disintegrating agent, lubricants and flavouring agent and compressed to form tablets.

COMPRESSION OF TABLETS

Granules are compressed to prepare tablets with the help of tablet-making machines which can be of following types :

1. Single-punch machines
2. Multi-punch machines
3. Rotary tablet machines
4. Double rotary tablet machines
5. Dry Cota tablet machines

1. Single punch machines

A single-punch machine generally consists of following parts :

1. Hopper — To store and supply the granules.
2. Hopper shoe — To supply granules to die.
3. Upper punch — For compression of granules.
4. Lower punch — For adjustment of capacity and to help in bringing the tablet out.
5. Ejection regulator — For ejection of tablet.
6. Capacity regulator — For adjustment of capacity.
7. Die — For compression of granules. It allows upper punch to come downward.

Working of single-punch tablet machine

When we start rotating the driving wheel several movements take place. These movements are as follows :

1. Upper punch comes to the upper most position and lower punch drops to the lowest position in the given adjustment.
2. Hopper shoe moves over the surface of die cavity and granules come from shoe to die.
3. Hopper shoe moves aside, upper punch comes down and compresses the granules to form a tablet. Lower punch remains stationary.
4. Upper punch goes up and lower punch also moves up and there is ejection of tablet and the cycle restarts.

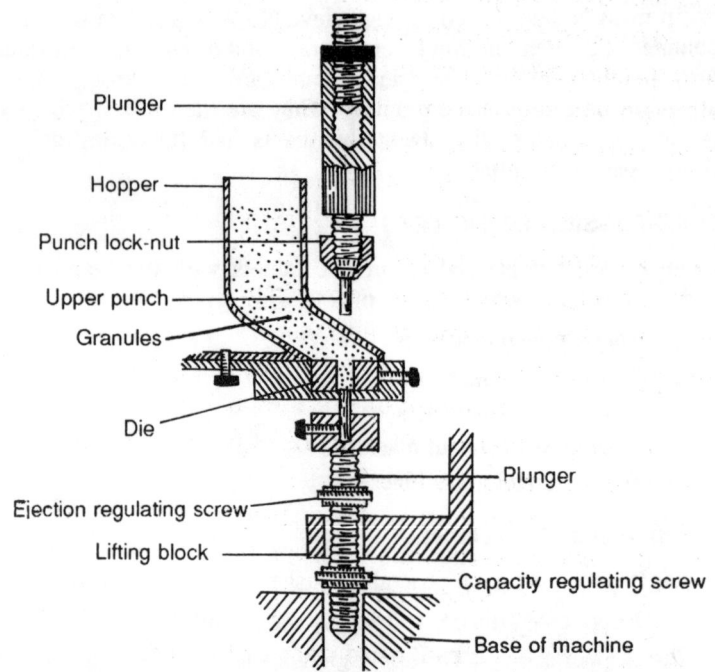

Fig. 12.1. Hand-operated single-punch tablet making machine.

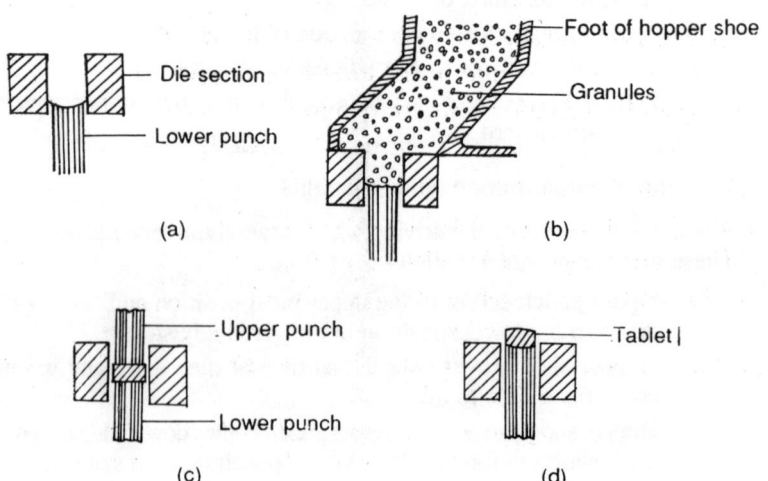

Fig. 12.2 (a, b, c & d). Steps involved in compression of granules into tablets.

2. **Multi-punch tablet machines**

Multi-punch tablet machine works on the same principle as that of single punch but in multi-punch tablet machine in one stroke we get number of tablets in more than one die provided in the machine.

3. **Rotary tablet machines**

Rotary tablet machines have about 70 sets of dies and punches which can produce up to 12,000 tab/min. These machines are used for large scale production. It consists of a rotating head having three parts :

1. An upper part consisting of upper punches;
2. Middle part having dies;
3. A lower part consisting of lower punches.

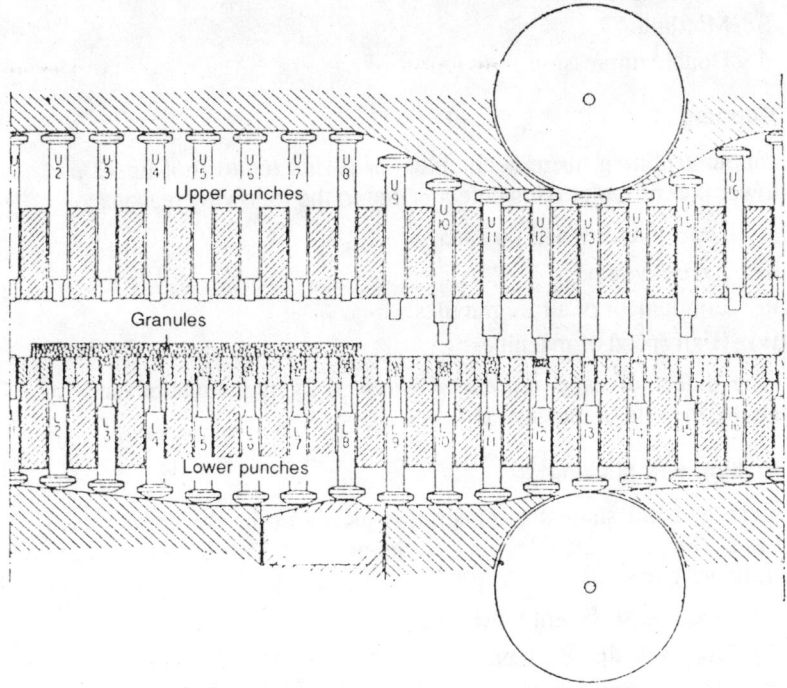

Fig. 12.3. Rotary tablet machine showing the compression cycle.

A large hopper supplies granules to the feed frame on movement of the head, the dies come under the feed frame in succession and are filled with granules. Compression takes place gradually by upper and lower punches and tablets are ejected out.

4. Double rotary tablet machines

Double rotary tablet machine means two rotary machines are assembled together. It consists of two rollers, two hoppers and two compression heads.

5. Dry Cota tablet machines

This machine consists of two rotary machines driven by single shaft. Core tablet is compressed by one machine and then it is transferred to second machine for compression coating.

Manufacturing Defects in Tablets

1. Capping
2. Picking and sticking
3. Mottling
4. Double impression

1. Capping

In capping/splitting, there is complete or partial removal of upper part or lower part of tablet. This defect is due to the following reasons :

  (i) Defective dies and punches;

 (ii) Excessive fines;

(iii) Entrapment of air in granules;

(iv) High speed of machine.

The defect of capping can be removed by regranulation and by changing the sets of dies and punches.

2. Picking and sticking

In picking, small amount of material is picked up by the upper punch and in sticking, the granules stick to the die wall. This defect is due to the following reasons :

  (i) Due to insufficient lubricant;

 (ii) Due to damp granules;

(iii) Use of worn out dies and punches.

The problem can be corrected by using dry granules, new set of dies and punches and optimum quantity of lubricant.

3. Mottling

This defect occurs when colour does not distribute evenly throughout the tablet. Mottling can be due to following reasons :

(i) Migration of dyes during drying process;

(ii) Due to difference of colours in drugs and additives.

4. Double impression

This defect occurs when monogram is printed on tablet. Lower punch has the monogram which gives impression on the tablet during compression. Sometimes, before ejection, lower punch gives unwanted upward movement and provides a second light impression on the tablet. This defect can be removed by correcting undesirable movement of the lower punch.

Tablet Coating

Purpose of coating

1. To prevent the exposure of medicament to atmospheric effect.
2. To make the tablet more elegant.
3. To improve unpleasant taste and odour of the drug.
4. To produce sustained release preparations.
5. To prevent the disintegration in stomach.

Methods of coating

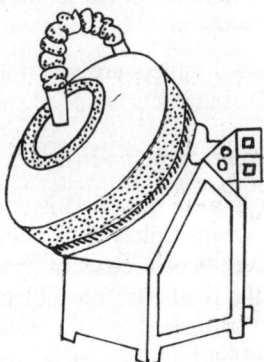

(i) Pan coating
    (a) Sugar coating
    (b) Film coating
    (c) Enteric coating

(ii) Press coating

(i) Pan coating

It is done in a pan made of copper or stainless steel. The coating is done in the pan which rotates with the help of an electric motor. Pan coating method is used for sugar coating, film coating, and enteric coating.

Fig. 12.4. Tablet coating pan.

(a) Sugar coating

The various stages of sugar coating process are as follows :

1. Sealing or water-proofing
2. Sub-coating
3. Smoothing

4. Colouring and finishing

5. Polishing

1. *Sealing or water-proofing*

In this step tablets are given one or two coatings of water-proof materials like shellac solution, cellulose acetate phthalate and silicones. This prevents the tablets from absorbing water when they come in contact with syrup. After sealing, tablets are removed from the pan and are dried completely for further coatings.

2. *Sub-coating*

Dried water-proof tablets are placed in pan which is then rotated. Subcoating solution (acacia + sugar) is gradually added. Tablets are allowed to rotate until they become sticky. Then sticky tablets are dusted with dusting powder (talc, starch, precipitated chalk, etc.). Rotation is continued until they lose their tendency to adhere each other.

Both the steps are repeated until the tablets are sufficiently covered and rounded. Precautions are taken to ensure that after every coating tablets are thoroughly dried.

3. *Smoothing*

Subcoated tablets are given few coatings of heavy syrup in a rotating pan. These tablets are dried simultaneously to achieve a smooth surface.

4. *Colouring and finishing*

The colouring of tablets is done by giving several coatings of coloured dilute syrups followed by coloured heavy syrups. Tablets are then dried and given 3 or 4 coats of syrup which provides elegance to the tablet. After the final coat, the tablets are again dried.

5. *Polishing*

Polishing is done in a canvas drum known as polishing pan. Dried tablets are placed in polishing pan. To this, solution of bees wax or any other suitable material is added. Volatile solvent evaporates with the formation of thin coating on tablets.

(b) **Film coating**

Film coating is generally given to tablets by dissolving polymer in some organic solvent and then spraying it over tablets in a rotating pan. They are later dried to form a permanent film. Advantages of film coating are as follows :

1. Time required is less.
2. Less labour is required.
3. Cost of production is less.
4. Water-proofing or sealing is not required.
5. Coating time is reduced.
6. Tablets of better strength are produced.
7. Increase in weight of tablet is insignificant.
8. Material cost is less.

(c) Enteric coating

There are some drugs which are required to disintegrate in intestine, and need to pass the stomach as such without any absorption. For such preparation, enteric coating is required. Enteric coating requires adjuvants like cellulose acetate phthalate, shellac solution, fatty acids, waxes, etc.

Enteric coating is done due to following requirements :

1. When the action is desired in intestines only.
2. For delayed action of medicament.
3. When drugs get decomposed in stomach due to acidic medium.
4. When drugs produce irritation is stomach.

(ii) Press coating or compression coating

This is also known as dry coating as this coating is done by compressing the dried granules over pre-compressed core tablet. The process is carried out in dry Cota rotary tablet machine.

Evaluation of Tablet

Following tests are carried out for production of good quality tablets :

1. Diameter, size and shape of tablet
2. Thickness of tablets
3. Uniformity of weight
4. Percentage of medicament
5. Rate of disintegration
6. Mechanical strength
7. Friability test

1. Diameter, size and shape of tablets

B.P. 1958 has specified the diameter of tablets between $\frac{6}{32}''$ to $\frac{20}{32}''$. All the tablets should have definite diameter and variation in diameter is allowed up to ±5%.

Tablets of various sizes and shapes are manufactured by manufacturers but generally they are circular with either flat or biconvex faces.

2. Thickness of tablet

All the tablets are allowed for thickness variation up to the limit of ±5% of the size of tablet. Thickness of tablet can be measured with the help of micrometer calipers. Thickness variation is due to the following reasons :

1. Difference of density of granules;
2. Compression pressure variation;
3. Change in speed of compression.

3. Uniformity of weight

It is desirable that all the tablets should have uniform weight. According to I.P. variation limits are prescribed and they shall fall within the prescribed limits.

Table 12.1. Weight variation limits

S. No.	Average weight	Percentage deviation in weight variation
1.	120 mg or less	±10
2.	More than 120 mg and less than 300 mg	±7.5
3.	300 mg or more	±5

This test is carried out for 20 tablets. Tablets are weighed individually and their average weight is calculated. If not more than two tablets fall outside the prescribed range the sample passes the test.

4. Percentage of medicaments

Percentage of medicament can be calculated by performing assay for the drug. Tablets are assayed according to the prescribed method given in pharmacopoeia. Average weight of medicament present in each tablet is calculated and compared with prescribed limits.

5. Rate of disintegration

This test is performed to calculate the time taken by the tablet to disintegrate. Different types of tablets require different rate of disintegration, e.g., chewable tablets which are dissolved slowly in mouth cavity need not comply disintegration test. While for oral tablets, rate of disintegration has to be within pharmacopoeial limits.

Disintegration test apparatus

It consists of two glass beakers in which a glass or plastic tube is fitted with rust-proof sieve No. 10 at the bottom. Water is placed in beakers which is thermostatically maintained at a temperature of 37°C (±2°C). Five tablets are placed in each tube and the motor is switched on. Guided disc over the tablets does not allow them to float and imparts a slight pressure on the tablets. The tubes are then allowed 30 up and down movements till all the tablets disintegrate and particles remain above the wire mesh.

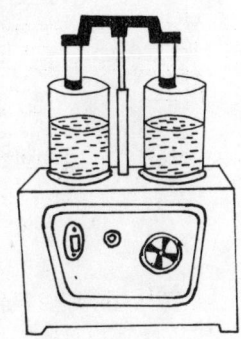

Fig. 12.5. Disintegration test apparatus.

6. Mechanical strength

Pharmacopoeia has not fixed any standards for mechanical strength. To check the hardness, manufacturers themselves adopted some devices. These are :

1. Monsanto hardness tester
2. Pfizer tablet hardness tester.

1. Monsanto hardness tester

It comprises of a spring which can be compressed by moving the screw knob. The tablet to be tested is placed in the provided space and the reading of indicator is adjusted to zero. Desired pressure is then applied by moving the screw knob in clockwise direction until the tablet breaks.

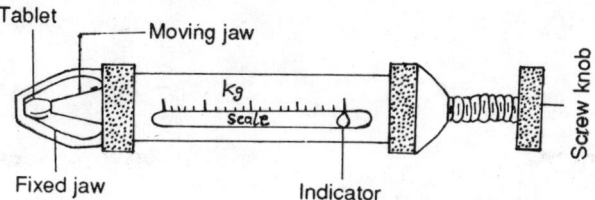

Fig. 12.6. Monsanto tablet hardness tester.

2. **Pfizer tablet hardness tester**

It has got similarity in its shape to that of a plier and works on its principle. The tablet to be evaluated is placed in between the jaws and pressure is applied with the help of handle until the tablet breaks. The reading on the dial corresponds to the pressure applied and is the hardness of the tablet.

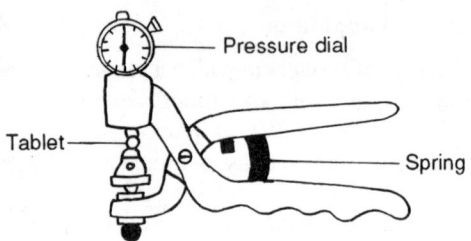

Fig. 12.7. Pizer tablet hardness tester.

7. **Friability test**

This test is done to check the ability of tablets to withstand the wear and tear during transportation. The apparatus used for this test is known as friabilator.

Friabilator consists of a plastic chamber having two parts which revolve at a speed of 25 r.p.m. Generally 20 tablets are weighed and placed in this chamber which is then rotated for 4 minutes (100 revolutions). The tablets are removed and weighed. Loss in weight indicates the friability. The tablets to be evaluated pass this test if the loss in weight is less than 0.8%.

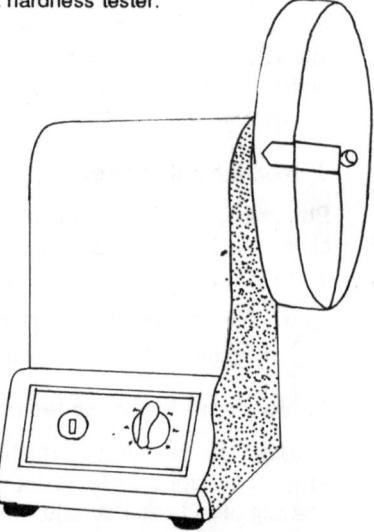

Fig. 12.8. Friabilator.

13

Capsules

Definition

Capsules are solid unit dosage forms in which the drug is enclosed in a soluble shell made of gelatin. Capsules are available as hard capsules and soft capsules. Hard capsules are used for filling solid substances whereas soft capsules are used for filling semi-solids and liquids.

Advantages

1. They are easy to administer because of their smooth and slippery nature.
2. Bitter and unpleasant taste can be masked by enclosing in a tasteless shell.
3. They are easy to handle and carry.
4. They are more attractive in appearance.
5. They provide ease in dispensing a single dose.

Disadvantages

1. They cannot be used for administration of extremely soluble materials, e.g., KCl, KBr, etc.
2. Hygroscopic drugs cannot be filled in capsules.
3. Concentrated solutions which require dilution before administration cannot be filled into capsules.

Hard Gelatin Capsules

They are used for administration of powders and other solid medicaments. The capsule shell is generally made of gelatin, titanium dioxide and colouring agent. Hard gelatin capsules consist of two parts, i.e., body and cap. Solid medicament is filled into body of the capsule and then cap is placed over it. They are available in various sizes designated by numbers varying from 000 to 5.

Properties of powdered drug to be filled in capsules

In order to achieve minimum weight variation and uniformity in finished product, following properties of powders must be considered :

Table No. 13.1. Approximate capacity and capsule number

Number	Capacity in mg
000	950
00	650
0	450
1	300
2	250
3	200
4	150
5	100

1. Flow properties of the powder

The powder must be free flowing in nature. Flow properties can be increased by adding substances like talc, stearic acid and magnesium stearate, etc.

2. Angle of repose

Angle of repose is a measurement of cohesiveness of the particles. It can be defined as the maximum angle which is formed between the surface of a pile of powder and horizontal surface. Powder flows very smoothly if the angle of repose is around 25-30°.

3. Hopper position

Hopper must be positioned properly so as to avoid uneven distribution of powder particles.

Hand operated capsule filling machine

This machine consists of following parts :
1. Frame having 200-300 holes
2. A loading tray
3. A powder tray
4. A peg plate having 200-300 pegs·
5. A lever
6. A cam handle
7. A sealing plate fitted with rubber top

Method of filling hard gelatin capsules

Loading tray containing empty gelatin capsules is placed over the frame. By operating cam handle, bodies and caps can be separated out. Now powder tray is placed in a proper position so that accurate quantity of powder can be filled with scraper. Peg plate is lowered down so as to press the filled powder downwards. Peg plate is raised and remaining quantity of powder is filled again in similar fashion with the help of scraper. After complete filling, powder tray is removed and the cap holding tray is placed in position. Sealing plate fitted with rubber top is now lowered and the lever is used to lock bodies and caps. Loading tray is removed and filled gelatin capsules are then collected.

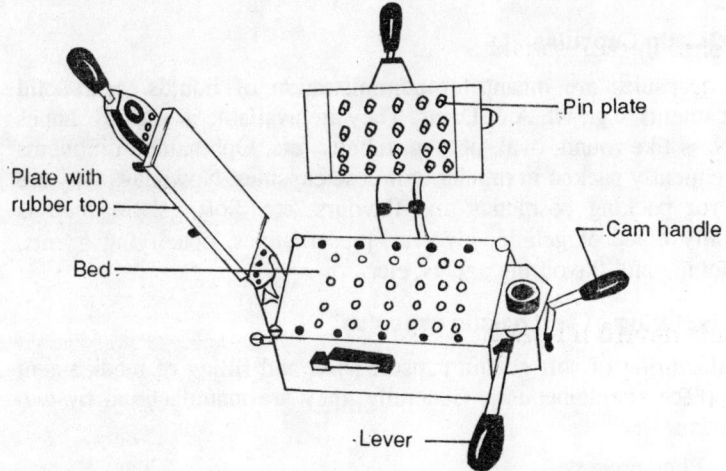

Fig. 13.1. Capsule filling machine (hand operated).

Cleaning and polishing of capsules

Capsules require following methods of dusting/polishing operations before bottling, stripping and labelling.

1. Salt polishing

Filled capsules are rotated in a tablet coating pan along with granular sodium chloride. The capsules are separated from salt by screening operation.

2. Cloth dusting

In this method capsules are individually rubbed with a soft cloth which may or may not be pregnant with oil. It gives a better gloss to the product.

3. Brushing

Here the capsules are put under rotating soft brushes which help to remove the dust from the capsule shell.

Sealing of capsules

Sealing or banding is done for three major purposes :

  (i)   To provide a distinctive appearance to the product.

  (ii) To prevent separation of capsules.

  (iii) To ensure that the medicament may not come out of the capsule during rough handling.

It is accomplished by banding with molten gelatin laid around the joint in a strip and dried.

Soft Gelatin Capsules

These capsules are meant for administration of liquids, semi-solid medicaments, e.g., vit. A & D, etc. They are available in various shapes and sizes like round, oval, oblong, tubular, etc. Ophthalmic ointments are frequently packed in tubular unit dose capsules. Nowadays they are used for packing cosmetics and flavours, etc. Soft gelatin shell is generally made of gelatin, glycerin, preservatives, opacifying agents, sweetening and flavouring agents, etc.

Manufacturing of soft gelatin capsules

Manufacturing of soft gelatin capsule shell and filling of medicament takes place simultaneously. Generally, they are manufactured by two methods :

  1. Plate process

  2. Rotary die process

1. Plate process

It consists of two plates, i.e., upper plate and lower plate. Warmed sheet of gelatin is placed over lower plate having number of cavities or moulds. The sheet is drawn into these cavities by applying vacuum. Then measured amount of liquid medicament is poured over it. Over this another sheet of gelatin is placed. Then upper plate is kept over it and pressure is applied to both the plates. Filled and sealed capsules are then cut into individual capsules by razor blades attached with moulds.

2. Rotary die process

This is an automatic machine in which two continuous sheets of gelatin are supplied to two die rolls rotating in opposite directions. As gelatin sheet comes in between the rollers, measured quantity of medicament to be filled is injected through a metering device. Heat and the pressure exerted by the die rolls seals the two halves together. The capsules are then washed with naphtha solution and dried.

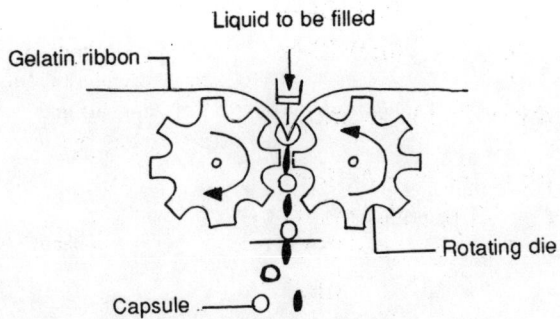

Fig. 13.2. Rotary machine.

Evaluation of Capsules

Various tests performed for standardization of capsules are as follows :

1. Weight variation test

Twenty filled hard gelatin capsules are taken at random and weighed individually. Their average weight per capsule is then calculated. The capsules pass the test if the weight of individual capsule falls within 90-110% of the average weight. If it does not meet this requirement then the weight of the contents of each individual capsule is determined and compared with the average weight of contents.

For soft gelatin capsules, shells are carefully opened by cutting and contents are removed by washing with suitable solvent. Shells are dried and weighed. Content weight of individual capsules is then calculated.

2. Contents uniformity test

This test is meant for all capsules used for oral administration. In this, assay is done as per individual monographs given in pharmacopoeia.

3. Disintegration test

In case of enteric coated capsules, this test is done to meet the prescribed requirements. One capsule is placed in each tube, which is then suspended in the beaker to move up and down for 30 minutes, unless otherwise stated in the monograph. The capsules pass this test if no residue of drug remains on the mesh of tubes.

Appendices

I

Drug Interactions

The term 'Drug interaction' can be defined as a change in response to drugs which sometimes occurs when two or more drugs are taken together. Sometimes it occurs when drugs are taken along with food and drinks which contain certain ingredients which interfere with the action of drug. Some commonly known drug interactions are given below.

S. No.	Name of drug	The drug in combination	Type of interaction
1.	Alcohol	Cimetidine	Blood alcohol levels are increased significantly when cimetidine is given concomitantly.
2.	Aspirin	Alcohol	It may increase the risk of gastrointestinal irritation and bleeding.
3.	Aspirin	Methotrexate	Aspirin may displace methotrexate from protein binding site thereby increasing its effect. Therefore dose of methotrexate must be monitored.
4.	Aspirin	Probenecid	Aspirin can antagonise the uricosuric effect of probenecid, therefore this combination should not be used.
5.	Allopurinol	Theophylline	Allopurinol decreases clearance of theophylline.
6.	Antacids	Bisacodyl	Bisacodyl tablets should not be taken within one hour of antacids or milk because premature disintegration of enteric coating occurs and release of drug in the stomach may cause irritation.
7.	Aluminium hydroxide	Famotidine	Aluminium hydroxide reduces both the rate and extent of absorption of famotidine but it has no effect when it is given after 2 hours.

Contd.

S. No.	Name of drug	The drug in combination	Type of interaction
8.	Amitriptyline	Diazepam, oxazepam, chlordiazepoxide, nitrozepam, benzodiazepines	Benzodiazepine provides a synergistic effect with amitriptyline. The combination is very fatal.
9.	Amitriptyline or impiramine	Antihypertensive substances except guanethidine and possibly clonidine	Antidepressant may cause a lowering of blood pressure and there may be an increased hypotensive effect; reduction in dosage of the antihypertensive is required.
10.	Amitriptyline or impiramine	Guanethidine	Tricyclic antidepressants antagonise the effect of guanethidine by blocking uptake into adrenergic nerve endings where it must be concentrated.
11.	Barbiturate or chloral hydrate, gluthemide	Alcohol	Excessive depression of CNS may result from combined use. So alcoholic beverages should be avoided along with it.
12.	Calcium salts	Phenobarbitone phenytoin	Anticonvulsant drugs reduce the absorption of calcium salts, therefore oral vitamin D should be supplemented along with anticonvulsants.
13.	Cholestyramine	Digoxin	Absorption of digoxin gets reduced by 30% - 40% when administered along with cholestyramine.
14.	Chlorpromazine, prochlorpromazine, haloperidol	Antacids	Use of an antacid containing magnesium trisilicate may decrease plasma level.
15.	Cimetidine	Aluminium magnesium hydroxide	Antacid reduces absorption of cimetidine therefore it should be administered one hour apart.

Contd.

S. No.	Name of drug	The drug in combination	Type of interaction
16.	Cimetidine	Morphine	Serious side-effects like apnoea, grandmal seizure, confusion, disorientation, may occur after 24 hours when morphine has already been used.
17.	Clemastine	Alcohol	Clemastine does not enhance CNS effects of alcohol.
18.	Cyclosporin	Diliazem	Combination of these two produces increase in blood concentration of cyclosporin and some of its metabolites. It may cause arthralgia.
19.	Dextro-propoxyphene	Warfarin	Action of warfarin is increased.
20.	Diazepam	Phenytoin	Plasma level and activity of phenytoin get increased.
21.	Digoxin, digitoxin	Barbiturates	Barbiturates accelerate metabolism of digitoxin, an increase in the dosage of latter is desired.
22.	Digoxin, digitoxin	Calcium preparation	Oral use of calcium preparation does not give appreciable response to digitalis glycosides but if calcium salts are given by I.V. route the effect is increased.
23.	Digoxin, digitoxin	Diuretics, potassium depleting (thiazide furosemide)	If potassium loss, as may be caused by a diuretic, remains uncorrected, the heart becomes more sensitive to the effects of digitalis. Approach is to use greater amounts of potassium-rich food.
24.	Digoxin	Diltiazem	Diltiazem reduces clearance of digoxin.
25.	Digoxin	Metoclopra-mide	When its solid dosage form is used, serum levels of digoxin are decreased.
26.	Digoxin	Quinidine	Significant reduction in digoxin serum level and therapeutic effects are observed when quinidine is withdrawn. Protein binding of digoxin is not affected by quinidine whereas both renal and non-renal clearance get halved.

Contd.

S. No.	Name of drug	The drug in combination	Type of interaction
27.	Digoxin	Quinidine and spironolactone	Quinidine and spironolactone decrease renal and non-renal clearances and provides prolonged digoxin plasma half-life. Therefore the dose of digoxin should be: reduced.
28.	Digoxin	Quinidine and verapamil	Additive effect of verapamil and quinidine are observed on the serum levels of digoxin.
29.	Erythromycin	Theophylline	Total clearance, terminal half-life volumes of distribution of erythromycin.
30.	Fluphenazine	Amitriptyline, nortriptyline, impramine, protriptyline	High doses of tricyclic antidepressants can increase plasma level of phenothiazines.
31.	Folic acid	Phenytoin	Use of phenytoin may lead to development of folic acid deficiency. If folic acid replacement therapy is necessary an increase in seizure frequency may result, possibly necessitating an adjustment of the dosage of phenytoin.
32.	Guanethidine	Alcohol	The effect of guanethidine is increased and there is greater risk of orthostatic hypotension therefore beverages should be avoided.
33.	Guanethidine	Amphetamine	In combination, amphetamine may decrease the effect of guanethidine.
34.	Hydrochlor thiazide	Indomethacin, sulindac	Indomethacin shows a rise in systolic blood pressure after two weeks.
35.	Isoniazid	Rifampicin	Combination of these two drugs may cause fulminant hepatitis.
36.	Insulin	Alcohol	Variable alterations in hypoglycemic responses are observed, depending upon the amount of alcohol consumed. Persons consuming large quantities of alcoholic beverages show severe hypoglycemia.

Contd.

S. No.	Name of drug	The drug in combination	Type of interaction
37.	Lithium salts	Sodium salts	High sodium intake increase, elimination of lithium. Extra care is required when effervescent preparations or sodium containing antacids are given.
38.	Magnesium hydroxide	Famotidine	Magnesium hydroxide reduces both the rate and extent of absorption of famotidine but has no such effect when taken two hours apart.
39.	Methotrexate	Naproxen	When given in combination serious adverse effects like death may occur.
40.	Methyl-phenytoin	Phenytoin	Plasma level and activity of phenytoin increases.
41.	Propranolol	Hypoglycemic agents like insulin, tolbutamide	Propranolol may increase the action of hypoglycemic agent with additional danger of β-adrenergic blocking action of propranolol.
42.	Propranolol	Quinidine	This combination produces decrease in the metabolism of β-blockers.
43.	Pheno-barbitone	Theophylline	Dose of theophylline should be increased by 30% when taken along with phenobarbitone.
44.	Phenytoin	Paracetamol	Toxicity of paracetamol increases in patients who are taking liver microsomal enzyme inducer such as alcohol or phenytoin. It requires management of toxicity of paracetamol.
45.	Phenytoin	Sodium valproate	Plasma levels of phenytoin get lowered but no effect on therapeutic action.
46.	Pyridoxine	Levodopa	Pyridoxine antagonises the action of levodopa by increasing its metabolism in the peripheral tissues. Patients on levodopa therapy should avoid multivitamins and other preparations containing pyridoxine.

Contd.

S. No.	Name of drug	The drug in combination	Type of interaction
47.	Potassium depleting diuretics	Hypoglycemic agents, insulin, tolbutamide	Diuretic may increase blood glucose levels and it requires an upward adjustment of dosage of hypoglycemic agent.
48.	Ranitidine	Alcohol	Blood alcohol levels significantly increase when ranitidine is given in combination.
49.	Coumarin, anticoagulants (warfarin, dicumarol)	Aspirin and other salicylates	Increased anticoagulant effect.
50.	Coumarin, anticoagulants (warfarin, dicumarol)	Barbiturates (pheno-barbitone, pento-barbitone)	Barbiturates increase the rate of metabolism of anticoagulants; decreased response to anticoagulants necessitates an increase in dosage.
51.	Coumarin, anticoagulants (warfarin, dicumarol)	Chlor-amphenicol	In combination, anticoagulant activities may be increased.
52.	Warfarin, dicumarin	Phenytoin	The effect of phenytoin may be increased and the action of anticoagulant decreases.
53.	Warfarin, dicumarol	Quinidine	Quinidine increases anticoagulant activity and then reduction in dosage of latter becomes necessary.
54.	Warfarin, dicumarol	Vitamin K	Vitamin K antagonises the action of the anticoagulants and has been used as an antidote in managing overdosage or excess responses to the latter.

II

Pharmaceutical Calculations

Q. 1. If the dose of phenobarbital for an adult is 15 mg. What will be the dose for a child of 8 years old according to Young's rule?

(Ans. 6 mg)

Q. 2. How will you dispense the following prescription?

Rx

Hyoscine hydrobromide   gr 1/150

M. ft. pulvis mitte tales quinque.

Hint :

  (a) 1 grain of drug + 24 grains of lactose

  (b) 1 grain of above mixture + 11 grains of lactose

Q. 3. Prepare 50 ml of normal saline solution.   **(Ans.** 0.45 g)

Q. 4. Prepare 1/2 fl. oz of 1% solution of gentian violet.

(Ans. 2.18 gr)

Q. 5. How will you dispense the following prescription?

Rx

Zinc oxide	20 g
Salicylic acid	2 g
Starch powder	78 g

M. ft. pulvis consperus mitte 10 g.

Q. 6. How will you dispense the following prescription?

Rx

Codeine phosphate   gr 1/6

M. ft. pulvis mitte tales tres.

Hint : 1 grain of drug + 11 grains of lactose

Q. 7. Prepare 1 pint solution of 60% alcohol from 90% alcohol.

(Ans. Vol. of 90% alcohol = 399 ml)

Q. 8. Prepare 2 fl oz of 1 : 5000 solution of potassium permanganate.

(Ans. 0.175 grain)

Q. 9. Prepare 50 ml of 2% solution of mercurochrome.   **(Ans.** 1 gm)

Q. 10. How will you prepare 1 fl. oz of 1 : 80 solution of zinc sulphate?

(Ans. 5.468 grains)

Q. 11. Prepare 8 fl. oz of sodium chloride so that 2 teaspoonfuls of it diluted to one quart will make 1 : 1000. **(Ans. 36.4 g)**

Q. 12. How will you dispense the following prescription?

Rx

Castor oil	8 ml
Aqua ad	25 ml

M. ft. emulsio mitte 25 ml.

Hint : O : W : G
          4 : 2 : 1
          8 : 4 : 2

Q. 13. Using Fried's rule calculate the dose for an 8-month old infant if average adult dose of a drug is 250 mg. **(Ans. 13.3 mg)**

Q. 14. In what proportion should 30% alcohol and 90% alcohol be mixed to make 20 ml of 50% alcohol?
(Ans. 30% alcohol = 13.3 ml; 90% alcohol = 6.7 ml)

Q. 15. Find the concentration of sodium chloride required to produce a solution iso-osmotic with blood plasma.

Given : mol. wt. of NaCl = 58.5; No. of ions = 2 **(Ans. 8.8 g/lt)**

Q. 16. Find the percentage of dextrose required to make 100 ml of isotonic solution. Dextrose is a non-ionising solute and its mol. wt. is 180. **(Ans. 5.4%)**

Q. 17. Using freezing point data calculate the concentration of sodium chloride to make 1% solution of cocaine hydrochloride iso-osmotic with blood plasma.

Freezing point of 1% w/v solution of cocaine HCl = –0.09°C

Freezing point of 1% w/v solution of sodium chloride = –0.576°C

(Ans. 0.746% w/v)

Q. 18. How will you dispense the following prescription?

Rx

Olive oil	4 ml
Aqua ad	30 ml

M. ft. emulsio mitte 100 ml.

Hint : O : W : G
          4 : 2 : 1
          8 : 4 : 2

Q. 19. How will you dispense the following prescription?

Rx

Turpentine oil	8 ml

Aqua ad   50 ml
M. ft. emulsio mitte 100 ml.
Hint :   O : W : G
              4 : 4 : 2
              8 : 8 : 4

Q. 20. How will you dispense the following prescription?
Rx
Liquid paraffin   3 ml
Aqua ad   30 ml
M. ft. emulsio mitte 60 ml.
Hint :   O : W : G
              3 : 2 : 1
              6 : 4 : 2

Q. 21. Prepare 600 ml of 60 percent alcohol from 95 percent alcohol.
                    (Ans. 379 ml to be diluted to 600 ml)

Q. 22. Prepare 250 ml of a solution of acetic acid containing 4 per cent real acetic acid.
Hint : Real acetic acid 33%   **(Ans. 30.3)**

Q. 23. How will you prepare 4 suppositories of zinc oxide each containing 2 grains of the drug, using cocoa butter as a base? Mould size is 15 gr and displacement value is 5.

   (Ans. For six suppositories : base = 87.6 grains; total wt. = 99.6 grains)

Q. 24. How will you dispense the following prescription?
   Rx
Dry ext. hammelis   gr ii
Olei theobromatis — quantitum sufficientum
Fiat suppositorium grana triginta mitte sex.
(Ans. For 8 suppositories : base = 229.4 grains; total weight = 245.5 grains)

Q. 25. Prepare 6 suppositories of bismuth subgallate containing 300 mg of the drug. Displacement value of bismuth subgallate is 3 and mould capacity is 1 g.
                    (Ans. For 8 suppositories : drug = 2.4 g; base = 7.2 g)

III

Revision Questions

Chapter 1. PRESCRIPTIONS

Q. 1. Translate the following Latin terms into English :

(i)	p.p.a.	(ii)	Coch. parv. h.s.s.
(iii)	s.o.s	(iv)	Mitte tales decem
(v)	Sig. o.m.s.	(vi)	b.d.s.
(vii)	m. ft. mist	(viii)	dol. urg
(ix)	Aq. ad	(x)	mod. dict. ut
(xi)	Rx	(xii)	ss
(xiii)	m.s.a.	(xiv)	p.r.n.
(xv)	b.t.i.d.	(xvi)	b.i.d.
(xvii)	sex. ind	(xviii)	o.m.
(xix)	o.n.	(xx)	i.e.
(xxi)	c.c.	(xxii)	pro singulis
(xxiii)	ana	(xxiv)	Hac. nocte

Q. 2. How much 90% v/v alcohol would be needed to make 5 litres of 50% v/v alcohol?

Q. 3. If 15 gm of a drug is dissolved in 2 litres of water, how many milligrams of the drug would be contained in each millilitre?

Q. 4. How many parts of 85%, 60%, 30% and 20% alcohol be mixed together to get 5 litres of 40% alcohol?

Q. 5. How will you prepare 1 pint of a 1 in 1000 solution?

Q. 6. Define the term prescription? What are the different parts of prescription?

Q. 7. Give the metric equivalence of :

(i)	1 drachm	(ii)	1 pint
(iii)	20 grains	(iv)	2 pints
(v)	10 fl. ounce	(vi)	4 drachm

Q. 8. How much water should be added to 250 ml of 5% w/v solution of a drug to make a solution such that 5 ml diluted to 500 ml will give 1 : 5000 solution?

Q. 9. Send 30 ml of potassium permanganate solution so that two 5 ml spoonful diluted to 500 ml will make 1 in 1000 solution.

Q. 10. Send 20 ml of 4% solution of potassium permanganate and label with direction for preparing 1 litre of 1 in 2500 solution.

Q. 11. How many ml of 0.1% w/v solution of mercury bichloride can be prepared from 50 tablets each containing 0.47 gm of drug?

Q. 12. Send 200 ml of 5% sodium chloride from 20% solution.

Q. 13. What is the percentage of zinc oxide in an ointment prepared by mixing 300 g of 7% ointment, 100 g of 5% ointment and 50 g of 5% ointment?

Q. 14. Required 1 pint of a 1 in 80 solution of zinc sulphate.

Q. 15. Required 4 oz of a solution so that 2 teaspoonful diluted to a pint makes 1 in 1000 solution.

Q. 16. Discuss various sources of errors while dispensing a prescription. How can they be corrected?

Q. 17. In what proportion should 12%, 8% and 3% alcohol be mixed to get 5% alcohol?

Chapter 2.   INCOMPATIBILITIES IN PRESCRIPTIONS

Q. 1. Classify incompatibility. Describe in detail various incompatibilities involving alkaloidal salts?

Q. 2. Differentiate between :

  (i)   Tolerated and adjusted incompatibility

  (ii) Therapeutic incompatibility and drug interaction.

Q. 3. Incompatible prescriptions :

  1. *Rx*

    Pot. permanganate   60 mg

    Liq. glucose q.s.

    Make pill, send 50.

  2. *Rx*

    Silver nitrate   0.1%

    Sodium chloride q.s.

    Water q.s. to make up to 20 ml.

    Send eye drops.

  3. *Rx*

    Liq. strych. hydrochlor   2 ml

    Spt amm aromat   1 ml

    Water ad 5 ml.

    Make mixture.

4. *Rx*

   Menthol   20
   Thymol   40
   Camphor   40
   Mag. carb. levis q.s.
   Make dusting powder.

5. *Rx*

   Aspirin   300 mg
   Water q.s.
   Make mixture, send 10 doses.

6. *Rx*

   Sodium sulphate   4 g
   Sodium bicarbonate   8 g
   Liq. ferric chloride   1 ml
   Aqua ad 180 ml.
   Ft. mistura, mitte talis 60 ml.

7. *Rx*

   Aminophylline   gr iss
   Sugar of milk   gr iii
   Ft. capsule mitte talis X.

8. *Rx*

   Liq. ferric chloride   1 ml
   Potassium iodide   2 g
   Potassium citrate   4 g
   Aqua ad 6 ml.
   Ft. mistura.

9. *Rx*

   Phenol   0.5 mg
   Menthol   0.1 g
   Tragacanth   0.5 g
   Olive oil   50   ml

10. *Rx*

    Glycerine boracis   30 ml
    Sodium bicarbonate   5 g
    Aqua ad 120 ml.
    Ft. collunarium.

11. *Rx*

| Terpin hydrate | 3.0 g |

Simple syrup ad 120 ml.
Ft. mist.

12. *Rx*

| Pot. chlorate | 4.0 g |
| Syp. ferric iodide | 15 ml |

Purified water ad 180 ml.
Ft. mist.

13. *Rx*

Cocaine hydrochloride	0.3 g
Boric acid	1.5 g
Sodium borate	1.2 g

Purified water ad 60 ml.

14. *Rx*

| Phenobarbitone sodium | 0.6 g |
| Ammonium bromide | 8.0 g |

Water to make 100 ml.
Make mixture.

15. *Rx*

| Chloral hydrate | 15.0 g |
| Sodium bromide | 11.25 g |

Elixir aromatic ad 60 ml.
Ft. mist.

16. *Rx*

| Tetracycline hydrochloride | 250 mg |
| Chalk | 50 mg |

M. ft. pulvis.

17. *Rx*

| Phenobarbital | 125 mg |

Elixir phenobarbital q.s. 15 ml.
M. ft. solutio.

18. *Rx*

Turpentine oil	25%
Soft soap	5%
Dil. acetic acid	5%

Purified water q.s.
Ft. linimentum.

19. *Rx*

Sodium salicylate	5 g
Lemon syrup	20 ml
Water ad 75 ml.	
Ft. mistura.	

20. *Rx*

Quinine hydrochloride	grain two
Sodium salicylate	drachm one
Aquam ad ounce three.	
Ft. mistura.	

Chapter 3. POSOLOGY

Q. 1. What is posology?

Q. 2. Discuss the methods for calculation of children's paediatric dosage.

Q. 3. Discuss the factors influencing the calculation of doses of medicine.

Q. 4. Calculate the dose for child if the adult dose is 60 mg and age of child is 6 yrs.

Chapter 4. POWDERS

Q. 1. Define the term 'powder' and classify them. How are powders containing minute quantities of potent medicaments compounded?

Q. 2. Describe the method of preparation of effervescent powders. What is a snuff?

Q. 3. What are the advantages and disadvantages of powders as unit dosage forms?

Q. 4. Justify the ingredients used in the effervescent granules with valid reasons.

Q. 5. Write short notes on eutectic mixtures.

Q. 6. How snuffs and dentifrices are formulated and prepared?

Q. 7. Classify powders. Describe the general method of dispensing powders containing eutectic combinations.

Q. 8. Differentiate between tablet triturates and cachets.

Q. 9. Write short notes on bulk powders for external use.

Chapter 5. MONOPHASIC LIQUID DOSAGE FORM

Q. 1. Describe the principles involved and techniques in enhancing solubility of drugs.

Q. 2. How will you prepare the following?

   (i) Lotions

   (ii) Throat paints

   (iii) Sprays

Q. 3. State general methods of preparation of

   (a) Diffusible and indiffusible mixture

   (b) Eye drops

Q. 4. Differentiate between

   (i) Douche and enema

   (ii) Lotion and liniment

   (iii) Gargles and mouth washes

   (iv) Syrups and elixirs

Q. 5. Discuss the importance of pH and isotonicity for preparation of eye drops? What are different methods to control isotonicity.

Chapter 6. BIPHASIC LIQUID DOSAGE FORM

Q. 1. Discuss the properties of suspended systems.

Q. 2. (a) What is a primary emulsion? (b) How can stable emulsion be prepared?

Q. 3. How will you establish whether an emulsion is o/w or w/o? Classify emulgents?

Q. 4. Define emulsions. How stability of emulsions can be improved?

Q. 5. Why all emulsions appear milky white?

Q. 6. Differentiate between the following :

   (i) Flocculated and deflocculated suspension

   (ii) Phase volume ratio and phase inversion

   (iii) O/w and w/o emulsion

   (iv) Creaming and sedimentation

   (v) Suspension and emulsion

Q. 7. What are emulsions? Give the wet gum and dry gum method for the preparation of emulsions. Give applications of emulsions.

Chapter 7.   OINTMENTS

Q. 1. Define an ointment. How does it differ from paste? What are the desirable properties of an ideal ointment base?

Q. 2. How is stainless iodine ointment prepared?

Q. 3. Differentiate between cream, ointment, paste and jellies.

Q. 4. Classify various bases used for ointments with their merits and demerits. Write a note on packing of ointments.

Q. 5. Discuss various factors governing selection of an ideal ointment base.

Chapter 8.   SUPPOSITORIES AND PESSARIES

Q. 1. Define displacement value? What are suppositories?

Q. 2. How will you prepare 6 suppositories (approx. 4 gm each) containing 25% of medicament having a displacement value of 2.0?

Q. 3. How are suppositories packed? Give method for finding out displacement value of a new substance.

Q. 4. Send 12 suppositories of tannic acid each weighing approximately 4 g and containing 300 mg of tannic acid (displacement value of tannic acid is 0.9).

Q. 5. Classify various bases used for suppositories with their merits and demerits. Which suppository base would you recommend for tropical countries?

Chapter 9.   DENTAL AND COSMETIC PREPARATIONS

Q. 1. What are dentifrices? Discuss the various ingredients, their uses and importance in preparation of such products.

Q. 2. Classify shampoos and give their specific uses. Discuss the additives used in their formulation.

Q. 3. Discuss the following :

   (i)   Antiperspirants and deodorants

  (ii)   Depilatories

 (iii)   Lipsticks

 (iv)   Various ingredients used in the formulation of cosmetic creams.

Chapter 10 & Chapter 11.   STERILE DOSAGE FORMS AND OPHTHALMIC PRODUCTS

Q. 1. Define sterility and give method for preparation of water for injection.

Q. 2. What are pyrogens? How are these removed while preparing water for injection?

Q. 3. Describe the tests for

   (i) Pyrogenicity

  (ii) Sterility

Q. 4. Find out the quantity of sodium chloride required to form a solution isotonic with blood plasma (mol. wt. of sodium chloride is 58.5 and dissociates into 2 ions).

Q. 5. Find out the proportion of glucose required to form a solution isotonic with blood plasma (mol. wt. of glucose is 180 and it is non-ionising).

Q. 6. Send 200 ml of 5% sodium chloride solution from 20% solution.

Q. 7. Define isotonicity and give specific gravity method for adjustment of isotonicity in parenteral solutions.

Q. 8. How much quantity of boric acid shall be required to prepare 100 ml of isotonic eye wash.

    Freezing point depression of 1% boric acid = –0.288°C

    Freezing point of blood plasma = –0.52°C

Q. 9. Calculate the amount of boric acid required to make 1% cocaine hydrochloride solution isotonic with tear secretion.

    Depression of freezing point due to 1% cocaine hydrochloride =
                                       –0.09°C

    Depression of freezing point due to 1% boric acid = –0.28°C

    Depression of freezing point due to blood = –0.52°C

Q. 10. Discuss various considerations involved in the development of formulae for parenteral products.

Q. 11. Discuss is detail evaluation of parenteral products.

Q. 12. Calculate the percentage of sodium chloride required to render 1.5% solution of cocaine hydrochloride isotonic with blood stream.

    Freezing point of 1% w/v solution of cocaine hydrochloride = –0.9°C

    Freezing point of 1% w/v solution of sodium chloride = –0.576°C

    Freezing point of blood = –0.52°C

Q. 13. What are the various sources of contamination in parenteral product.

Chapter 12. TABLETS

Q. 1. Discuss the various tests which are generally done to maintain the quality control of tablets.

Q. 2. (a) Write the various methods of preparation of granules from the powdered drug. (b) Describe the common defects which can occur in compressed tablets.

Q. 3. Write short notes on

   (a) Friability test

   (b) Disintegration test

   (c) Common defects of compressed tablets

   (d) Excipients used in tablet formulation

Q. 4. Why tablets are still considered to be the formulation of choice among oral preparations? Write the various methods of granulation.

Q. 5. Discuss in detail :

   (i) Properties of tablets

   (ii) Pan coating and press coating of tablets

   (iii) Manufacturing defects in tablets

Q. 6. Give methods for coating of tablets.

Q. 7. Differentiate between disintegration test and dissolution test.

Chapter 13.   CAPSULES

Q. 1. Differentiate between hard gelatin capsules and soft gelatin capsules. Give a brief account of their method of preparation.

Q. 2. Give a brief account of soft gelatin capsule. Discuss the filling and sealing machine for soft gelatin capsule.

Q. 3. Write short notes on

   (a) Hard gelatin capsule

   (b) Soft gelatin capsule

   (c) Angle of repose

Q. 4. Differentiate between hard and soft capsules.

IV

Patent and Proprietary Products of Some Common Ailments

1. ANTACIDS

1. **Acigon**   Boehringer-Mannheim
   Aluminium hydroxide gel   80   mg
   Alginic acid   0.2   g
   Mag. trisilicate   40   mg
   Sodium bicarbonate   70   mg
         Chewable tablets   (Rs. 2.39/10 tabs)

2. **Aludrox**   Wyeth
   Dried aluminium hydroxide gel   840 mg
         Tablets   (Rs. 9.42/50 tabs)
         Suspension   (Rs. 13.43/3.50 ml)

3. **Digene gel**   Boots
   Aluminium hydroxide gel   830 mg
   Methyl polysiloxane   25 mg
   Mag. hydroxide   185 mg
   Sod. carboxy methyl cellulose   100 mg   .
         Suspension   (Rs. 13.18/200 ml)

4. **Diovol Forte tabs**   Wallace
   Alum. hydroxide gel   300 mg
   Mag. hydroxide   250 mg
   Activated dimethicone   40 mg
         Tablets   (Rs. 2.65/10 tabs)

5. **Gelusil**   Warner
   Alum. hydrox. gel   250 mg
   Mag. trisilicate   500 mg
         Tablets   (Rs. 1.45/10 tabs)
         Suspension   (Rs. 13.78/400 ml)

6. **Polycrol Forte gel**   Nicholas Piramal
   Alum. hydrox. gel   5 g
   Mag. hydrox.   100 mg
   Activated dimethicone   125 mg

Suspension (Rs. 143.25/200 ml)
Tablets (Rs. 4.02/10 tabs)

7. **Riflux liquid** SOL
   Alum. hydrox. gel   300 mg
   Sod. alginate   200 mg
   Mag. trisilicate   125 mg
   Suspension (Rs. 16.60/200 ml)
   Tablets (Rs. 66/20 × 6 tabs)

8. **Rolac Plus** Wyeth
   Megaldrate   480 mg
   Dimethicone   20 mg
   Tablets (Rs. 5.70/10 tabs)

2. LAXATIVES AND PURGATIVES

1. **Cremaffin** Boots
   Milk of magnesia   11.25 ml
   Liquid paraffin   3.75 ml
   Emulsion (Rs. 22/200 ml)

2. **Dulcolax** German Remedies
   Bisacodyl   5 mg
   Tablets (Rs. 49.50/10 × 10 tabs)

3. **Julax** Rallis
   Bisacodyl   10 mg
   Casanthranol   10 mg
   Tablets (Rs. 94.15/10 × 10 tabs)

4. **Pursennid** Sandoz
   Senna glycosides   18 mg
   Dioctyl sod. sulfosuccinate   50 mg
   Tablets (Rs. 5.86/10 tabs)

5. **Cremaffin FS** Boots
   Isapgol husk   3.5 g/14.25 g
   Powder (Rs. 30/100 g)

3. ANTIDIARRHOEALS

1. **Amibex NA** Swift
   Nalidixic acid   300 mg
   Metronidazole (as benzoate)   200 mg
   Tablets (Rs. 17.95/10 tabs)

2. **Dependal M** Eskayef
   Furazolidone   100 mg
   Metronidazole (as benzoate)   300 mg
                 Tablets (Rs. 5.57/10 tabs)

3. **Flagyl F** Rhone-Poulenc
   Metronidazole   400 mg
   Furazolidone   100 mg
                 Tablets (Rs. 10.56/10 tabs)

4. **Furoxone** Eskayef
   (a) **Furoxone tablets**
   Furazolidone   100 mg
                 Tablets (Rs. 2.27/10 tabs)

   (b) **Furoxone suspension**
   Furazolidone   35.7 mg
   Pectin   75   mg
   Light kaolin   1   g/ml
                 Suspension (Rs. 7.24/50 ml)

5. **Imodium** Ethnor
   Loperamide hydrochloride   2 mg
                 Capsules (Rs. 2.85/4)

6. **Imosec S** Ethnor
   Loperamide hydrochloride   2 mg
   Streptomycin sulphate   500 mg
                 Capsules (Rs. 11.89/4)

7. **Kaolin with Neomycin** Abbott
   For 15 ml
   Kaolin   3 g
   Pectin   65 mg
   Neomycin sulphate   150 mg
                 Suspension (Rs. 12.07/60 ml)

8. **Lomotil** Searle
   Diphoxylate hydrochloride   2.5 mg
   Atropine sulphate   0.25 mg
                 Tablets (Rs. 1.88/10)

9. **Lopamide** Torrent
   Loperamide HCl   2 mg
                 Tablets (Rs. 4.90/10)

10. **Sporlac** Uni-Sankyo
    Spores of lactobacillus sporogenes 60 million
                        Tablets (Rs. 8.19/10)
11. **Tini-F suspension** Kopran
    For 5 ml
    Tinidazole   100 mg
    Furazolidone   35 mg
                        Suspension (Rs. 11.99/50 ml)
12. **Walamycin suspension** Wallace
    For 5 ml
    Colistin sulphate   12.5 mg
                        (Rs. 17/30 ml)

4. ANTIHYPERTENSIVE DRUGS

1. **Amlogard** Pfizer
   Amlodisine (as besylate)   5 mg & 10 mg
                        Tablets (5 mg — Rs. 262.95/10)
2. **Angiopril** Torrent
   Captopril   25 mg & 50 mg
                        Tablets (25 mg — Rs. 26.80/10)
                                (50 mg — Rs. 51.60/10)
3. **Atacardil** Sun Pharma
   Atenolol   50 & 100 mg
                        Tablets (50 mg — Rs. 18.38/10)
                                (100 mg — Rs. 35.18/10)
4. **Betacard** Torrent
   Atenolol   50 mg & 100 mg
                        Tablets (50 mg — Rs. 12.90/10)
                                (100 mg — Rs. 24.56/10)
5. **Betaloc** Astra-IDL
   Metoprolol tartrate   50 mg & 100 mg
                        Tablets (50 mg — Rs. 9.17/10)
                                (100 mg — Rs. 16.85/10)
6. **Calaptin** Boehringer-Mannheim
   Verapamil   40 mg & 80 mg
                        Tablets (40 mg — Rs. 7.60/10)
                                (80 mg — Rs. 14.86/10)

7. **Cipril** Cipla
   Lisinopril

   2.5, 5 & 10 mg
   Tablets (2.5 mg — Rs. 20/10)
   (5 mg — Rs. 35/10)
   (10 mg — Rs. 60/10)

8. **Depin** Cadila
   Nifedipine

   10 mg & 5 mg
   Capsules (10 mg — Rs. 20.70/30)
   (10 mg — Rs. 66/100)
   (5 mg — Rs. 24/50)
   (5 mg — Rs. 29.80/100)

9. **Diltime-SR** Alidac
   Diltiazem HCl

   90 mg & 120 mg
   Tablets (90 mg — Rs. 37/10)
   (120 mg — Rs. 49/10)

10. **Envas** Cadila
    Enalapril maleate

    2.5, 5, 10 & 20 mg
    Tablets (2.5 mg — Rs. 9.50/10)
    (5 mg — Rs. 16.20/10)
    (10 mg — Rs. 30.70/10)
    (20 mg — Rs. 60.60/10)

11. **Lasix** Hoechst
    Frusemide

    40 mg
    Tablets (Rs. 80.85/25 × 10)

12. **Lipril** Lupin
    Lisinopril

    2.5 mg, 5 mg & 10 mg
    Tablets (2.5 mg — Rs. 15.35/10)
    (5 mg — Rs. 28.25/10)
    (10 mg — Rs. 58.45/10)

13. **Myogard - LA** Searle
    Nifedipine

    20 mg
    (Rs. 9.75/10)

5. ANALGESIC, ANTIPYRETICS AND NON-STEROIDAL ANTI-INFLAMMATORY AGENTS

1. **Beserol** Win-Medicare
   Paracetamol   450 mg
   Chlormezanone   100 mg
   Tablets (Rs. 23.64/10)

2. **Calpol** Burroughs Wellcome
   Paracetamol   500 mg
                                  (Rs. 2.95/10)
3. **Crocin** Duphar-Interfran
   Paracetamol   500 mg
                          Tablets (Rs. 3/10)
4. **Disprin** Reckitt & Colman
   Aspirin   350 mg
   Cal. carb   105 mg
   Anhydr. citric acid   35 mg
                          Tablets (Rs. 2.14/10)
5. **Dolac** Cadila
   Ketorolac tromethamine   10 mg
                          Tablets (Rs. 17.70/10)
5. **Fortwin** Ranbaxy
   Pentazocine (as lactate)   30 mg/1 ml inj.
                       Injection (Rs. 6.56/1 ml)
                          Tablets (25 mg — Rs. 21.91/12)
7. **Ketanov** Ranbaxy
   Ketorolac tromethamine   30 mg/ml inj.
                   Injection (Rs. 9.80/1 ampoule)
8. **Micropyin** Nicholas-Piramal
   Acetyl salicylic acid (microfined) 350 mg
   Caffeine   20 mg
                          Tablets (Rs. 2.16/10)
9. **Proxyvon** Wockhardt
   Dextropropoxyphene HCl   65 mg
   Acetaminophen   400 mg
                       Capsules (Rs. 8.05/8)
10. **Zimalgin** Rallis
    Analgin   250 mg
    Paracetamol   250 mg
    Caffeine   15 mg
    Codeine phosphate   5 mg
                          Tablets (Rs. 4.77/10)
11. **Brufen** Boots
    Ibuprofen   200 mg, 400 mg & 600 mg
                   Tablets (200 mg — Rs. 3.67/10)

$$(400 \text{ mg} - \text{Rs. } 6.51/10)$$
$$(200 \text{ mg} - \text{Rs. } 9.44/10)$$

12. **Bufex** CFL
    Ibuprofen   400 mg
    Paracetamol   500 mg
                        Tablets (Rs. 10/10)

13. **Butacortindon** Indon
    Oxyphenbutazone   100 mg
    Analgin   250 mg
                        Tablets (Rs. 5.75/10)

14. **Combiflam** Roussel
    Ibuprofen   400 mg
    Paracetamol   325 mg
                        Tablets (Rs. 8.39/10)

15. **Diclogesic** Torrent
    Diclofenac sod.   50 mg
    Paracetamol   500 mg
                        (Rs. 2.77/10)

16. **Diclomax 25/50** Torrent
    Diclofenac sod.   25 & 50 mg
                    Tablets (25 mg — Rs. 5.50/10)
                             (50 mg — Rs. 9.90/10)

17. **Diclonac** Lupin
    Diclofenac sod.   50 mg
                        Tablets (Rs. 7.09/10)

18. **Emflam Plus** Merck
    Ibuprofen   400 mg
    Paracetamol   325 mg
                        Tablets (Rs. 8.17/10)

19. **Nac-50** Systopic
    Diclofenac sod.   50 mg
                        Tablets (Rs. 7.17/10)

20. **Relaxyl tablets** Franco-Indian
    Diclofenac sod.   50 mg
                        Tablets (Rs. 6.85/10)

21. **Systaflam** Systopic
    Acetaminophen   650 mg
    Dextropropoxyphene HCl   32.5 mg

Oxyphenbutazone   100   mg
                        Tablets (Rs. 14/10)
22. **Voveran**   Hindustan Ciba-Geigy
Diclofenac sodium   50 mg
                        Tablets (Rs. 70.90/10 × 10)

6. SEDATIVES AND TRANQUILISERS

1. **Alzolam**   Sun Pharma
Alprozolam   0.25 mg, 0.5 mg & 1 mg
                        Tablets (0.25 mg — Rs. 6.46/10)
                                 (0.5 mg — Rs. 11.94/10)
                                 (1 mg — Rs. 16.58/10)

2. **Alzopax**   LA Pharma
Alprozolam   0.25 mg, 0.5 mg & 1 mg
                        Tablets (0.25 mg — 6.18/10)
                                 (0.5 mg — Rs. 10.50/10)
                                 (1 mg — Rs. 15.76/10)

3. **Anatensol injection**   Sarabhai
Fluphenazine de canoate   25 mg per ml
                        Injection (Rs. 27.82/1 ml vial)

4. **Atarax**   Uni-UCB
Hydroxyzine HCl   10 mg & 25 mg
                        Tablets (10 mg — Rs. 6.15/10)
                                 (25 mg — Rs. 9.80/10)

5. **Calmpose**   Ranbaxy
Diazepam   2, 5 & 10 mg
                        Tablets (5 mg — Rs. 8/10)

6. **Hexidol**   Torrent
Haloperidol   1.5 mg
Trihexyphenidyl HCl   1.5 mg
                        Tablets (Rs. 6.01/10)

7. **Larpose**   Cipla
Lorazepam   1 mg
                        Tablets (Rs. 6/10)

8. **Librium**   Roche
Chlordiazepoxide   10 mg
                        Tablets (Rs. 5.45/10)

9. **Restyl** Protec
   Alprozolam   0.25 mg, 0.5 mg & 1 mg
                              Tablets (0.25 mg — 6.25/10)
                                       (0.5 mg — Rs. 11.49/10)
                                       (1 mg — Rs. 14.64/10)

10. **Valium** Roche
    Diazepam   5 mg
                              Tablets (Rs. 6.85/10)

7. ANTI-EMETICS AND ANTI-NAUSEANTS

1. **Avomine** Rhone-Poulenc
   Promethazine theoclate   25 mg
                              Tablets (Rs. 2.06/4)
                                       (Rs. 6.62/10)

2. **Domperon** Alidac
   Domperidone   10 mg
                              Tablets (Rs. 16.70/10)

3. **Domstal** Torrent
   Domperidone   10 mg
                              Tablets (Rs. 15.90/10)

4. **Maxeron-MPS** Wallace
   Metoclopramide HCl   5 mg
   Activated dimethicone   125 mg
                              Tablets (Rs. 7.55/10)

5. **Perinorm** IPCA
   Metoclopramide HCl   10 mg
                              Tablets (Rs. 4.60/10)
                                       (Rs. 95/250)

6. **Reglan** CFL
   Metoclopramide monohydrochloride 10 mg
                              Tablets (Rs. 4/10)
                              Injection (Rs. 5.00/5 ml)

8. ANTIBIOTICS

1. **Anclox** Walter Bushnell
   Ampicillin (as trihydrate)   250 mg
   Cloxacillin (as sod.)   250 mg
                              Capsules (Rs. 40.80/8)

2. **Ampiryn** Cipla

Ampicillin   500 mg per vial
                    Injection (Rs. 5.42/5 ml vial)
3. **Ampoxin 500** Unichem
Ampicillin   250 mg
Cloxacillin   250 mg
                    Capsules (Rs. 49.90/10)
4. **Bacipen** Alembic
Ampicillin (as trihydrate)   250 mg & 500 mg
                    Capsules (250 mg — Rs. 9.04/4)
                              (500 mg — Rs. 16.78/4)
5. **Baxin** Lyka
Ampicillin (as trihydrate)   250 mg
Cloxacillin (as sod.)   250 mg
                    Capsules (Rs. 39.08/8)
6. **Betaspore** Aristo
Cephalexin   250 mg & 500 mg
                    Capsules (250 mg — Rs. 17.88/4)
                              (500 mg — Rs. 33.32/4)
7. **Bilactam dry syrup** CFL
For 5 ml
Ampicillin   125 mg
Cloxacillin   125 ml
                              (Rs. 23.35/30 ml)
8. **Biocilin** Biochem
Ampicillin trihydrate   250 mg & 500 mg
                    Capsules (Rs. 16.95/40 ml)
9. **Bluceff-P** Blue Cross
Cephalexin   125 mg
                    Tablets (Rs. 22.80/10)
10. **Campicillin** Cadila
Ampicillin   250 mg & 500 mg
                    Capsules (250 mg — Rs. 25.36/10)
                              (500 mg — Rs. 47.92/10)
11. **Ceff** Lupin
Cephalexin   250 mg & 500 mg
                    Tablets (250 mg — Rs. 18.16/4)
                             (500 mg — Rs. 31.74/4)

12. **Flemiclox** Mejda
    Amoxycillin   250 mg
    Cloxacillin   250 mg
                    Capsules (Rs. 30.03/6)
13. **Mox** Gufic
    Amoxycillin   250 mg & 500 mg
                    Capsules (250 mg — Rs. 7.74/3)
                              (500 mg — Rs. 14.22/3)
                              (Rs. 67.04/15)
14. **Novamox** Cipla
    Amoxycillin   250 mg & 500 mg
                    Capsules (250 mg — Rs. 39.23/15)
                              (250 mg — Rs. 15.77/6)
                              (Rs. 29.97/6)
                    Dry syrup (Rs. 11.26/30 ml)
                              (Rs. 19.46/60 ml)
15. **Penplus** Systopic
    Ampicillin (as trihydrate)   250 mg
    Cloxacillin (as sod.)   250 mg
    Lactobacillus sporogenes   60 million spores
                    Capsules (Rs. 35.38/6)

9. ANTI-TUBERCULAR DRUGS

1. **Combutol** Lupin
   Ethambutol HCl   200 mg, 400 mg, 600 mg,
                                        800 mg & 1000 mg
                    Tablets (200 mg — Rs. 5.15/10)
                            (400 mg — Rs. 9.54/10)
                            (600 mg — Rs. 13.76/10)
                            (800 mg — Rs. 18.11/10)
                            (1000 mg — Rs. 22.47/10)
2. **Mycobutol** Cadila
   Ethambutol   200 mg, 400 mg, 600 mg
                                        & 800 mg
                    Capsules (200 mg — Rs. 5.15/10)
                             (400 mg — Rs. 9.54/10)
                             (600 mg — Rs. 13.76/10)
                             (800 mg — Rs. 18.11/10)

3. **Rimactane** Hindustan Ciba-Geigy
   Rifampin   150 mg & 300 mg (caps) &
                                               450 mg (tabs)
                        Capsules (150 mg — Rs. 226.25/25 × 4)
                                  (300 mg — Rs. 414.75/25 × 4)
                        Tablets   (450 mg — Rs. 468.40/10 × 8)

4. **Rinizide** Lupin
   Rifampin   150 mg
   Isoniazide   100 mg
   Pyrazinamide   375 mg
                        Capsules (Rs. 31.82/10)

5. **Tibirim** Ranbaxy
   Rifampin   150 mg, 300 mg & 450 mg
                        Capsules (150 mg — Rs. 138.60/10)
                                  (300 mg — Rs. 10.66/4)
                                  (450 mg — Rs. 11.70/3)

10. ANTI-AMOEBIC DRUGS

1. **Flagyl** Rhone-Poulenc
   Metronidazole   200 mg & 400 mg
                        Tablets   (200 mg — Rs. 3.80/10)
                                  (400 mg — Rs. 6.34/10)

2. **Metrogyl** Unique
   Metronidazole   200 mg & 400 mg
                        Tablets   (200 mg — Rs. 3.62/10)
                                  (400 mg — Rs. 6.03/10)

3. **Asistogyl Plus** Aristo
   Metronidazole   400 mg
   Diloxanide furoate   500 mg
   Dimethicone   100 mg
                        Tablets   (Rs. 15.33/10)

4. **Entamizole** Boots
   Diloxanide furoate   250 mg
   Metronidazole   200 mg
                        Tablets   (Rs. 3.84/6)

5. **Qugyl** Searle
   Di-iodohydroxyzine   325 mg
   Metronidazole   250 mg
                        Tablets   (Rs. 11.12/10)

6. **Tinibid-DS** Crosslands
   Tinidazole   1000 mg
                                   Tablets (Rs. 7.75/2)
7. **Zil** Sarabhai
   Tinidazole   300 mg & 600 mg
                      Tablets (300 mg — Rs. 12.40/10)
                              (600 mg — Rs. 22.52/10)

11. ANTI-MALARIALS

1. **Emquin** Merck
   Chloroquine (as phosphate)   150 mg
                           Tablets (Rs. 7.97/12)
                           Syrup (Rs. 8.30/60 ml)
2. **Nivaquine** Rhone-Poulenc
   Chloroquine sulphate   200 mg
                           Tablets (Rs. 8.05/10)
                                   (Rs. 480/1000)
3. **Lariago** IPCA
   Chloroquine (as phosphate)   150 mg
                           Tablets (Rs. 9.70/12)
                    Suspension (Rs. 10.17/60 ml)
                       Injection (Rs. 2.68/5 ml)
4. **Rimodar** AFD
   Sulphadoxine   500 mg
   Pyrimethamine   25 mg
                           Tablets (Rs. 3.83/2)
5. **Stadmed** La-Quin
   Chloroquine (as phosphate)   250 mg
                           Tablets (Rs. 3.20/10)
                       Injection (Rs. 1.64/5 ml)
                          Liquid (Rs. 9.73/60 ml)

12. ANTI-HELMINTICS

1. **Bendex** Protec
   Albendazole   400 mg
              Chewable tablets (Rs. 7.88/10)
                    Suspension (Rs. 10.11/10 ml)

2. **Mebazole** Torrent
   Mebendazole   100 mg
                          Tablets (Rs. 3.60/6)
3. **Mebex** Cipla
   Mebendazole   100 mg
                          Tablets (Rs. 6.94/6)
4. **Pyramoate tabs** Franco-Indian
   Pyrantel (as parmoate)   250 mg
                          Tablets (Rs. 7.71/3)
5. **Vermisol** Khandelwal
   Levamisole   50 mg & 150 mg
                          Tablets (50 mg — Rs. 1.70/1)
                                   (150 mg — Rs. 2.70/1)
6. **Zentel** Eskayef
   Albendazole   400 mg
                          Tablets (Rs. 9.75/1)
                       Suspension (Rs. 12.70/10 ml)

13. ANTI-ASTHMATICS

1. **Asmapax Depot** Nicholas-Piramal
   Ephedrine (as resinate)   50 mg
   Theophylline   65 mg
   Phenobarb   30 mg
                          Tablets (Rs. 5.71/10)
2. **Asthalin** Cipla
   Salbutamol   2 mg & 4 mg
                          Tablets (2 mg — Rs. 3.31/10)
                                   (4 mg — Rs. 5.00/10)
                            Syrup (Rs. 10.90/112 ml)
                          Inhaler (Rs. 64.30/200 metered doses)
3. **Asthalin Rotacaps - Rotahaler** Cipla
   Salbutamol (as sulph)   200 mcg
                          Rotacaps (Rs. 38.58/30 rotacaps)
4. **Becoride** Glaxo Allenbury
   Beclomethasone dipropionate   100 mcg per actuation
                  Aerosol inhaler (Rs. 220/200 actuations)
5. **Bronchoplus** Biddle Sawyer
   Salbutamol   2 mg

Anhydrous theophylline   100 mg
                          Tablets (Rs. 4.15/10)
                          Syrup (Rs. 14.95/100 ml)

6. **Codiphylate** Cadila
   Theophylline ethanoate of piperazine 250 mg
                          Tablets (Rs. 28.95/100)
                          Elixir (Rs. 12.50/100 ml)

7. **Deriphyllin**   German Remedies
   For 2 ml
   Etophylline   169.4 mg
   Theophylline   50.6 mg
                          Ampoule (Rs. 2.12/2 ml)
                          Tablets (Rs. 2.25/10)
                          Syrup (Rs. 10.25/100 ml)

8. **Fintal Inhaler**   Rallis
   Sod. cromoglycate   1 mg
                          Inhalation (Rs. 119.70/can of 200 inhalations)

9. **Theolong** SOL
   Theophylline anhydrous   100 mg & 200 mg
         Sustain release capsules (100 mg — Rs. 77.50/10 × 10)
                                    (200 mg — Rs. 100.70/10 × 10)

10. **Vent** Kopran
    Salbutamol   2 mg
    Theophylline anhydrous   100 mg
                          Tablets (Rs. 146.78/10 × 3)
                          Liquid (Rs. 17.62/100 ml)

11. **Ventorlin**   Glaxo-Pharma
    Salbutamol (as salbutamol sulph)   4 mg & 8 mg
               Controlled release (4 mg — Rs. 6.28/10)
                          Capsule (8 mg — Rs. 9.04/10)

14. ANTI-ALLERGIC DRUGS

1. **Atarax** Uni-UCB
   Hydroxyzine HCl   10 mg & 25 mg
                          Tablets (10 mg — Rs. 6.15/10)
                                    (25 mg — Rs. 9.80/10)

2. **Avil, 25/50** Hoechst
   Pheniramine maleate   22.5 mg & 45 mg
                        Tablets (25 mg — Rs. 1.35/10)
                                 (50 mg — Rs. 1.92/10)

3. **Benadryl** Parke-Davis
   Diphenhydramine HCl   25 mg (caps) &
                                       50 mg (kapseals)
                        Capsules (Rs. 4.30/10)
                        Kapseals (Rs. 12.74/50)
                        Syrup (Rs. 12/114 ml)

4. **Incidal** Bayer
   Mebhydrolin napadicylate   76 mg (50 mg base)
                        Tablets (Rs. 2.91/10)

5. **Phenargan** Rhone-Poulenc
   Promethazine HCl   10 mg & 25 mg
                        Tablets (10 mg — Rs. 1.21/10)
                                 (25 mg — Rs. 1.87/10)
                        Elixir (Rs. 9.37/125 ml)

6. **Terfed** Cipla
   Terfenadine   60 mg
                        Tablets (Rs. 22.65/10)
                        Suspension (Rs. 19.74/50 ml)

7. **Trexyl** Ranbaxy
   Terfenadine   60 mg
                        Tablets (Rs. 23.05/10)
                        Suspension (Rs. 21.40/50 ml)

8. **Vallergan** Rhone-Poulenc
   Trimephrazine tartarate   10 mg
                        Tablets (Rs. 6.39/10)

15. ANTI-DIABETIC DRUGS

1. **Chlorformin** Cadila
   Chlorpropamide   50 mg
   Phenformin HCl   25 mg
                        Tablets (Rs. 2.90/10)

2. **Daonil** Hoechst
   Glibenclamide   5 mg
                        Tablets (Rs. 26.95/10 × 10)

3. **Diabinese** Pfizer
   Chlorpropamide   100 mg & 250 mg
                        Tablets (100 mg — Rs. 2.65/10)
                                 (250 mg — Rs. 4.19/10)

4. **Glyciphage** Franco-Indian
   Metformin HCl   0.5 mg
                        Tablets (Rs. 6.31/10)

5. **Human Noridsulin** Boots
   Highly purified neutral insulin   40 IU per ml
                        Vial (Rs. 159.80/10 ml vial)

6. **Insulatard** Boots
   Highly purified isophane insulin (NPH)
   Porcine   40 IU per ml injection
                        Injection (Rs. 102.88/10 ml vial)

7. **Insulin Zinc (Lentel)** Boots
   A mixture of 3 parts of insulin zinc suspension (amorphous) and
   7 parts of insulin zinc suspension (crystalline) prepared from
   bovin pancreas.
                        Injection (40 u — Rs. 30.60/10 ml)
                                   (80 u — Rs. 54.55/10 ml)

8. **Nordisulin** Boots
   Highly purified neutral insulin (porcine) 40 IU/ml
                        Injection (Rs. 102.70/10 ml vial)

16. ORAL CONTRACEPTIVES

1. **Ovral** Wyeth
   Di-Norgestrel   0.5 mg
   Ethinyl estradiol   0.05 mg
                        Tablets (Rs. 16.56/21)

2. **Ovral - L** Wyeth
   Norgestrel   0.33 mg
   (Equivalent to levonorgestrel 0.15 mg)
   Ethinyl estradiol   0.03 mg
                        Tablets (Rs. 12.29/21)

3. **Primovlar - 30** German Remedies
   Norgestrel   0.5 mg
   Ethinyl estradiol   0.03 mg
                        Tablets (Rs. 10/21)

4. **Triquilar**   German Remedies
   First 6 tabs
   Levonorgestrel   50 mg
   Ethinyl estradiol   30 mcg
   Next 5 tabs
   Levonorgestrel   75 mcg
   Ethinyl estradiol   40 mcg
   Next 10 days
   Levonorgestrel   125 mcg
   Ethinyl estradiol   30 mcg
                      Memo pack   (Rs. 15.50)

Index